Disclaimer

Medicine and nursing are continuously changing practices. The author and publisher have reviewed all information in this book with resources believed to be reliable and accurate and have made every effort to provide information that is up to date with best practices at the time of publication. Despite our best efforts we cannot disregard the possibility of human error and continual changes in best practices the author, publisher, and any other party involved in the production of this work can warrant that the information contained herein is complete or fully accurate. The author, publisher, and all other parties involved in this work disclaim all responsibility from any errors contained within this work and from the results from the use of this information. Readers are encouraged to check all information in this book with institutional guidelines, other sources, and up to date information. For up to date disclaimer information please visit: http://www.nrsng.com/about.

NCLEX®, NCLEX®-RN ®are registered trademarks of the National Council of State Boards of Nursing, INC. and hold no affiliation or support of this product.

Photo Credits:

All photos are original photos taken or created by the author or rights purchased at Fotolia.com. All rights to appear in this book have been secured. Some image rights were obtained via ECGpedia.com.

Some images within this book are either royalty-free images, used under license from their respective copyright holders, or images that are in the public domain. Images used under a creative commons license are duly attributed, and include a link to the relevant license, as per the author's instructions. All Creative Commons images used under the following license. All works in the public domain are considered public domain given life of the author plus 70 years or more as required by United States law.

140 Must Know Meds
Demolish Nursing Pharmacology

Nursing Assessment
Head-to-Toe Physical Assessment in Pictures

LAB VALUES
63 Must Know Labs for Nurses

Nursing Mnemonics
94 Memory Tricks to Demolish Nursing School

NRSNG.com | NursingStudentBooks.com

Jon Haws RN CCRN

First Kindle Edition 2015

Table of Contents

Your Free Gift!

As a way of saying thanks for your purchase, I'm offering a free PDF download:

"63 Must Know NCLEX® Labs"

With these charts you will be able to take the 63 most important labs with you anywhere you go!

You can download the 4 page PDF document by going to NRSNG.com/labs

How to use this book:

This book is divided into two sections; individual medications and medication classes. Under the individual medications you will find the most important information you need to know about the given medication to pass tests and provide safe patient care. This **is not to be considered** a complete list of all considerations for the medications but simply a guide to help you learn the MOST important tested information. The medication class section covers some of the most often tested medication classes and should be used to learn the general basics of some of the most common classes.

Introduction

I remember my first day as a sophomore nursing student in Nursing Pharmacology. To say I was lost is an understatement. It was like some one had dropped me off in a completely foreign land with an incomprehensible language. When I entered nursing school the only real health care experience I had was working as a transporter in a large hospital. Pharmacology was new to me and I was terrified that I would never be able to grasp the lingo.

The good news was my study partner had actually attended pharmacy school in India before coming to the United States to study nursing. The bad news was the **Pharmacology makes up about 15% of the questions on the NCLEX®** and I only had a semester to learn it!

The next few months were spent intently studying and taking practice exams. During the course of taking countless practice exams I would jot down every medication that was tested. I also would jot down the fact about the specific medication or class that was being tested.

This book is a compilation of the 140 must know meds for the NCLEX® and Nursing Pharmacology. These medications were the most tested. While the nursing considerations listed are not complete (and are not intended to be) they contain the most frequently tested material that you need to know for a given medication.

If you can learn the key facts about these medications you will ace your course and the NCLEX. The fact that you have downloaded this book proves that you are serious about your nursing career!

Oh yeah! I did end up passing Nursing Pharmacology with an "A" and continue to study pharmacology . . . but now I really enjoy it.

Happy Nursing!

-Jon Haws RN CCRN

NRSNG.com | NursingStudentBooks.com | SIMCLEX.com | Med of the Day Podcast

Alteplase

Generic Name

alteplase

Trade Name

t-PA

Indication

MI, acute ischemic stroke, occluded central lines

Action

converts plasminogen to plasmin which degrades the fibrin found in clots

Therapeutic Class

thrombolytics

Pharmacologic Class

plasminogen activators

Nursing Considerations

- contraindicated in active bleeding
- monitor closely for signs of bleeding (petechiae)
    - q 15 min X1hr
    - q 15-30 min X 8 hr
- use caution with patient who have had recent surgery
- may cause intracranial hemorrhage
- monitor for anaphylaxis
- use caution with uncontrolled hypertension
- assess neuro status during therapy

Atorvastatin

Generic Name

atorvastatin

Trade Name

Lipitor

Indication

management of high cholesterol (hypercholesterolemia), primary prevention of cardiovascular disease

Action

lowers total cholesterol as well as LDL while slightly increasing HDL. Inhibits HMG-CoA reductase which plays a role in the liver in cholesterol formation

Therapeutic Class

lipid-lowering agent

Pharmacologic Class

HMG-CoA reductase inhibitor

Similar Medications

simvistatin (Zocor), rosuvastatin (Crestor)

Nursing Considerations

- contraindicated in active liver disease
- may cause rhabdomyolysis
- monitor renal function
- monitor serum cholesterol before, about 4 weeks after starting, and frequently during drug therapy
- monitor liver function tests

- instruct patient to report muscle weakness (sign of rhabdomyolysis)

Acetaminophen

Generic Name

acetaminophen

Trade Name

Tylenol

Indication

pain, fever

Action

inhibit the synthesis of prostaglandins which play a role in transmission of pain signals and fever response

Therapeutic Class

antipyretic, non-opioid analgesic

Nursing Considerations

- do not exceed 4g of acetaminophen per day to limit risk for liver, renal, and cardiac damage
- overdose will lead to hepatotoxicity
- Acetadote is the antidote for overdose
- may increase risk for bleed with warfarin therapy
- may alter blood glucose measurements

Acyclovir

Generic Name

acyclovir

Trade Name

Zovirax

Indication

genital herpes, herpes zoster, chicken pox

Action

interferes with viral DNA synthesis

Therapeutic Class

antiviral

Pharmacologic Class

purine analogues

Nursing Considerations

- may cause seizures, renal failure, Stevens-Johnson syndrome, thrombotic thrombocytopenic purpura syndrome, diarrhea, dizziness, nausea
- monitor renal panel during administration
- assess lesions
- instruct patient to use proper protection during sexual intercourse

Albuterol

Generic Name

albuterol

Trade Name

Proventil

Indication

bronchodilator used to prevent airway obstruction in asthma and COPD

Action

binds to Beta2 adrenergic receptors in the airway leading to relaxation of the smooth muscles in the airways

Therapeutic Class

bronchodilator

Pharmacologic Class

adrenergic

Nursing Considerations

- may decrease the effectiveness of Beta Blockers
- use caution with
    - heart disease
    - diabetes
    - glaucoma
    - seizure disorder
- overuse of inhalers can lead to bronchospasm
- monitor for chest pain and palpitations
- can decrease digoxin levels

Alendronate

Generic Name

alendronate

Trade Name

Fosamax

Indication

osteoporosis (aging, menopause, corticosteroid induced)

Action

inhibits osteoclast activity leading to inhibition of resorption of bone

Therapeutic Class

bone resorption inhibitor

Pharmacologic Class

biphosphnates

Nursing Considerations

- take first thing in the morning with full glass of water 30 min prior to eating
- assess serum calcium and vitamin D
- may lead to muscle pain

Alprazolam

Generic Name

Alprazolam

Trade Name

Xanax

Indication

anxiety, panic disorder, manage symptoms of PMS, insomnia, mania, psychosis

Action

works in CNS to produce anxiolytic effect causing CNS depression.

Therapeutic Class

antianxiety agent

Pharmacologic Class

benzodiazepine

Nursing Considerations

- use caution with existing CNS depression, sleep apnea, renal dysfunction, hepatic dysfunction.
- may cause CNS depression, drowsiness, lethargy
- may lead to physical dependence, may experience tolerance effect
- assess anxiety and mental status
- Flumazenil is the antidote for overdose
- Grapefruit juice may increase blood levels

Amiodarone

Generic Name

Amiodarone

Trade Name

Cordarone

Indication

ventricular arrhythmias, SVT, ACLS protocol for v-fib and vTACH

Action

prolongs action potential, inhibits adrenergic stimulation, slows rate, decreases peripheral vascular resistance causing vasodilation

Therapeutic Class

Antiarrhythmic class III, Potassium channel blocker

Pharmacologic Class

none

Nursing Considerations

- may lead to ARDS, pulmonary toxicity, CHF, bradycardia, hypotension
- increases risk for QT prolongation
- increases digoxin levels
- increases activity of warfarin
- monitor EKG continuously while on therapy
- assess for signs and symptoms of ARDS
- monitor liver function test
- check dosage with another RN
- teach pt to monitor pulse daily and report abnormalities
- avoid drinking grapefruit juice

Amitryptiline

Generic Name

Amitryptiline

Trade Name

Elavil

Indication

depression, anxiety, insomnia

Action

increases effect of serotonin and norepinephrine in the CNS, exhibits anticholinergic effects

Therapeutic Class

antidepressant

Pharmacologic Class

tricyclic antidepressant

Nursing Considerations

- contraindicated in MI, heart failure, **QT prolongation**, glaucoma
- may increase risk for suicidal ideation
- may cause arrhythmias, hypotension, EKG changes
- may cause alterations in blood glucose levels
- may lead to general sedation and lethargy
- **do not use within 2 weeks of MAOIs**
- Instruct pt to take medication exactly as instructed
- monitor for orthostatic hypotension
- may lead to photosensitivity, instruct patient to use sunscreen
- may turn urine blue/green color.

Amlodipine

Generic Name

Amlodipine

Trade Name

Norvasc

Indication

hypertension, angina

Action

blocks transport of calcium into muscle cells inhibiting excitation and contraction

Therapeutic Class

antihypertensive

Pharmacologic Class

Ca channel blocker

Nursing Considerations

- may cause gingival hyperplasia
- grapefruit juice may increase drug level
- monitor blood pressure and pulse prior to and during therapy
- monitor intake and output
- assess for signs of CHF
- assess characteristics of angina
- instruct patient of interventions for hypertension and how to take blood pressure

Amoxicillin

Generic Name

amoxicillin

Trade Name

Moxatag

Indication

skin infections, respiratory infections, sinusitis, endocarditis prophylaxis, lime disease

Action

Inhibits synthesis of bacterial cell wall leading to cell death.

Therapeutic Class

anti-infectives, antiulcer agent

Pharmacologic Class

aminopenicillins

Nursing Considerations

- Contraindicated with penicillin allergy
- may cause seizures
- assess for rash, anaphylaxis
- excreted by kidneys - monitor renal labs
- monitor patient for diarrhea - bloody stool should be reported immediately

Ampicillin

Generic Name

Ampicillin

Trade Name

Principen

Indication

skin infections, soft tissue infections, otitis media, sinusitis, respiratory infections, GU infections, meningitis, septicemia

Action

bactericidal, broader spectrum than penicillin, binds to cell wall leading to bacterial cell death

Therapeutic Class

anti-infective

Pharmacologic Class

aminopenicillin

Nursing Considerations

- contraindicated in penicillin allergy, use caution in renal insufficiency
- may lead to seizures, diarrhea, anaphylaxes, super infection
- assess for infection
- monitor liver function tests
- instruct patient on signs of super infection: fury over growth on tongue, vaginal itching, loose and foul smelling stool
- pt should not use with oral contraceptive use.

Aspirin

Generic Name

Aspirin

Trade Name

Bayer Aspirin

Indication

rheumatoid arthritis, osteoarthritis, ischemic stroke and MI prophylaxis

Action

inhibits the production of prostaglandins which leads to a reduction of fever and inflammation, decreases platelet aggregation leading to a decrease in ischemic diseases

Therapeutic Class

antipyretics, non-opioid, analgesics

Pharmacologic Class

salicylates

Nursing Considerations

- use caution in bleeding disorders, chronic alcohol use
- may lead to Stevens-Johnson syndrome, laryngeal edema, and anaphylaxis
- increases risk for bleeding with warfarin, heparin, and clopidogrel
- increased risk for GI bleeding with NSAID use
- monitor liver function tests
- concurrent use with alcohol may increase risk for GI bleeding

Atenolol

Generic Name

atenolol

Trade Name

Tenormin

Indication

hypertension, angina, prevention of MI

Action

blocks the stimulation of $beta_1$ receptors in the SNS with minimal effect on $beta_2$ receptors

Therapeutic Class

antianginal, antihypertensive

Pharmacologic Class

beta blocker

Nursing Considerations

- Contraindicated in CHF, pulmonary edema, cardiogenic shock, bradycardia, heart block
- monitor hemodynamic parameters (HR, BP)
- May cause bradycardia, CHF, pulmonary edema
- Masks symptoms associated with diabetes mellitus
- advise to change positions slowly to prevent orthostatic hypotension
- instruct patient on how to take blood pressure

Atropine

Generic Name

atropine

Trade Name

Atro-pen

Indication

decreases oral and respiratory secretions, treats sinus bradycardia and heart block, treatment of bronchospasm

Action

Atropine is an anticholinergic which means that it inhibits the effects of the parasympathetic nervous system, specifically acetylcholine. This inhibition causes increase in HR, bronchodilation, decreased GI and respiratory secretions.

Therapeutic Class

antiarrhythmic

Pharmacologic Class

anticholinergic, antimuscarinic

Nursing Considerations

- Avoid in acute hemorrhage, tachycardia, and angle closure glaucoma
- monitor patient for tachycardia and palpitations
- may cause urinary retention in elderly patients
- patients may experience constipation due to slowed GI motility

Azithromycin

Generic Name

azithromycin

Trade Name

Zithromax

Indication

URI, chronic bronchitis, lower respiratory infections, otitis media, skin infections, various STIs, prevention of bacterial endocarditis, treatment of cystic fibrosis

Action

inhibits bacterial protein synthesis

Therapeutic Class

agents for atypical mycobacterium, anti-infectives

Pharmacologic Class

Macrolide

Nursing Considerations

- may lead to pseudomembranous colitis, pain, diarrhea, nausea, Stevens-Johnson syndrome, angioedema
- may increase risks for warfarin toxicity
- monitor patient for signs of anaphylaxis
- instruct patient to notify physician for diarrhea, or blood or pus in stool
- instruct patient to take medication exactly as prescribed

Benzotropine

Generic Name

benzotropine

Trade Name

Cogentin

Indication

treatment for Parkinson's disease

Action

anticholinergic properties in the CNS to reduce rigidity and tremors

Therapeutic Class

Antiparkinson agent

Pharmacologic Class

Anticholinergic

Nursing Considerations

- may lead to arrhythmias, hypotension, palpitations, and tachycardia
- anticholinergic effects like constipation, dry mouth
- assess for extrapyramidal symptoms
- instruct patient to take as directed
- instruct patient to maintain good oral hygiene

Biscodyl

Generic Name

biscodyl

Trade Name

Ducolax

Indication

treatment of constipation, bowel regimen

Action

stimulates peristalsis leads to fluid accumulation in the colon

Therapeutic Class

laxatives

Pharmacologic Class

stimulant laxatives

Nursing Considerations

- may lead to hypokalemia
- may cause abdominal pain and cramps
- use caution with milk
- assess for abdominal distention and bowel function
- instruct patient to drink 1500-2000 mL/day during therapy
- monitor fluid and electrolyte levels
- instruct patient to take as ordered

Bismuth Subsalicylate

Generic Name

Bismuth Subsalicylate

Trade Name

Kaopectate, Pepto-Bismol

Indication

diarrhea, heartburn, indigestion, H. pylori associated ulcer

Action

Stimulates the absorption of fluids and electrolytes in the intestinal wall, reduction in hypermotility of the stomach, and binds to toxins.

Therapeutic Class

antidiarrheal, antiulcer

Pharmacologic Class

adsorbant

Nursing Considerations

- contraindicated in aspirin hypersensitivity
- increase risk for impaction with geriatric and pediatric patients
- monitor liver profile
- bismuth may interfere with radiologic exams

Bupropion

Name

bupropion

Trade Name

Wellbutrin

Indication

depression, smoking cessation, treat ADHD in adults

Action

Therapeutic Class

Antidepressants, smoking deterrents

Pharmacologic Class

aminoketones

Nursing Considerations

- may lead to seizures, suicidal thoughts
- do not administer if patient is taking MAOI
- use caution with renal and liver impairment
- assess mental status
- instruct patient to avoid alcohol while taking bupropion

Buspirone

Generic Name

bupropion

Trade Name

Wellbutrin

Indication

management of anxiety

Action

relieves anxiety by binding to dopamine and serotonin receptors

Therapeutic Class

Antidepressants, smoking deterrents

Pharmacologic Class

aminoketones

Nursing Considerations

- do not administer concurrently with MOAI or grapefruit juice
- may lead to dizziness, drowsiness, fatigue, and weakness
- patient may experience chest pain, palpitations, tachycardia
- instruct patient to take as directed
- instruct patient to avoid alcohol and other CNS depressants

Butorphanol

Generic Name

Butorphanol

Trade Name

Stadol

Indication
moderate to severe pain, labor pain, sedation

Action

alters perception and response to pain by biding to opiate receptors in CNS

Therapeutic Class

Opioid Analgesic

Pharmacologic Class

opioid agonists/antagonists

Nursing Considerations

- use caution with concurrent use of MAOIs
- may cause confusion, hallucinations, sedation
- monitor for CNS depression
- assess blood pressure pulse and respirations during administration
- administer slowly through IV line

Calcium acetate

Generic Name

Calcium acetate

Trade Name

PhosLo

Indication

treatment of hypocalcemia, prevention of post menopausal osteoporosis, treatment of hypokalemia and hypomagnesaemia, adjunct in cardiac arrest, control of hyperphosphatemia with ESRD

Action

calcium is essential for nervous muscular and skeletal systems, helps maintain cell membranes, aids in transmission of nerve impulses and muscle contraction, aids in blood formation and coagulation

Therapeutic Class

mineral and electrolyte replacements/supplements

Pharmacologic Class

antacids

Nursing Considerations

- may cause cardiac arrest and arrhythmias
- phlebitis at site of insertion
- monitor hemodynamics
- may causes hypotension, bradycardia, and arrhythmias
- hypercalcemia can increase risk for digoxin toxicity
- administer slowly
- instruct pt on foods that contain Vitamin D and encourage adequate intake.
- monitor parathyroid hormone

Calcium carbonate

Generic Name

Calcium carbonate

Trade Name

Tums / Rolaids

Indication

treatment of hypocalcemia, prevention of post menopausal osteoporosis, treatment of hypokalemia and hypomagnesaemia, adjunct in cardiac arrest, used as antacid

Action

calcium is essential for nervous muscular and skeletal systems, helps maintain cell membranes, aids in transmission of nerve impulses and muscle contraction, aids in blood formation and coagulation

Therapeutic Class

mineral and electrolyte replacements/supplements

Pharmacologic Class

antacids

Nursing Considerations

- may cause cardiac arrest and arrhythmias
- monitor hemodynamics
- may causes hypotension, bradycardia, and arrhythmias
- hypercalcemia can increase risk for digoxin toxicity
- instruct pt on foods that contain Vitamin D and encourage adequate intake.
- monitor parathyroid hormone

Captopril

Generic Name

captopril

Trade Name

Capoten

Indication

hypertension, management of CHF, decrease progression of DM neuropathy

Action

block conversion of angiotensin I to angiotensin II, increases renin levels and decreases aldosterone leading to vasodilation

Therapeutic Class

antihypertensives

Pharmacologic Class

ACE Inhibitor

Nursing Considerations

- can cause neutropenia - check WBCs regularly
- use cautiously with potassium supplements and potassium sparing diuretics.
- use cautiously with diuretic therapy
- administer 1 hour before meals
- monitor blood pressure often
- monitor weight and fluid status
- monitor renal profile
- monitor CBC frequently
- May lead to Rhabdomyolysis
- Dry cough

Carbamazepine

Generic Name

carbamazepine

Trade Name

Tegretol

Indication
seizures, DM neuropathy, pain associated with trigeminal neuralgia

Action

affects Na channels in neurons leading to decreased synaptic transmission

Therapeutic Class

Anticonvulsant

Pharmacologic Class

none

Nursing Considerations

- interferes with oral contraceptives

- do not use with MAOIs
- may cause suicidal thoughts
- may cause Stevens-Johnson syndrome, agranulocytosis, aplastic anemia, thrombocytopenia
- do not consume grapefruit juice while taking this medication
- monitor CBC and platelet count
- monitor serum blood levels of medication often.

Carbidopa/levodopa

Generic Name

carbidopa/levodopa

Trade Name

Sinemet

Indication

Parkinson's disease

Action

levodopa is converted to dopamine and works as a neurotransmitter and carbidopa prevents the destruction of levodopa

Therapeutic Class

Antiparkinson agent

Pharmacologic Class

Dopamine Agonist

Nursing Considerations

- may cause orthostatic hypotension
- may cause dark urine
- weeks to months to take effect
- do not use with MAOIs
- don't use with glaucoma, melanoma
- assess for parkinsonian symptoms
- instruct patient to take as directed

Cefaclor

Generic Name

cefaclor

Trade Name

Ceclor

Indication
treatment of respiratory tract infections, skin infections, otitis media

Action

bacteriacidal, binds to bacterial cell wall causing cell death

Therapeutic Class

anti-infectives

Pharmacologic Class

Cephalosporin 2nd generations

Nursing Considerations

- contraindicated in cephalosporin and possibly penicillin allergies
- may need lead to seizures, pseudomembranous colitis, diarrhea, phlebitis at IV site, anaphylaxis
- Assess infection and allergies
- obtain cultures prior to therapy
- monitor bowel function
- may lead to super infection

Cefdinir

Generic Name

cefdinir

Trade Name

Omnicef

Indication

treatment of skin infections, otitis media

Action

bactericidal, binds to bacterial cell wall causing cell death

Therapeutic Class

anti-infectives

Pharmacologic Class

Cephalosporin 2nd generations

Nursing Considerations

- contraindicated in cephalosporin and possibly penicillin allergies
- may need lead to seizures, pseudomembranous colitis, diarrhea, phlebitis at IV site, anaphylaxis
- Assess infection and allergies
- obtain cultures prior to therapy
- monitor bowel function
- monitor for bleeding
- may lead to super infection

Celecoxib

Generic Name

celecoxib

Trade Name

Celebrex

Indication

osteoarthritis, rheumatoid arthritis, acute pain

Action

decreases pain and inflammation by inhibiting synthesis of prostaglandins

Therapeutic Class

antirrheumatics/NSAID

Pharmacologic Class

none

Nursing Considerations

- use caution with cardiovascular disease
- increases risk for MI, CVA, thrombosis
- may cause GI bleeding, Stevens-Johnson syndrome, dermatitis
- notify provider for new-onset abdominal pain or black stool

Cephalexin

Generic Name

cephalexin

Trade Name

Keflex

Indication

skin infections, pneumonia, UTI, otitis media

Action

bactericidal: binds to bacterial cell wall leading to cell death

Therapeutic Class

anti-infectives

Pharmacologic Class

Cephalosporin 1st generations

Nursing Considerations

- contraindicated with cephalosporin and serious penicillin allergies.
- may need lead to seizures, pseudomembranous colitis, diarrhea, phlebitis at IV site, anaphylaxis
- Assess infection and allergies
- obtain cultures prior to therapy
- monitor bowel function
- may lead to super infection
- may cause elevated liver enzymes

Chlorpromazine

Generic Name

chlorpromazine

Trade Name

Thorazine

Indication
second line treatment of schizophrenia and psychosis, nausea/vomiting, pre-op sedation, acute intermittent porphyria, headache, bipolar

Action

exhibits anticholinergic activity, alters effects of dopamine in CNS

Therapeutic Class

Antipsychotic, antiemetic

Pharmacologic Class

phenothiazines (dopamine D2 receptor antagonist)

Nursing Considerations

- may cause neuroliptic malignant syndrome, sedation, tardive dyskineisa, hypotenstion, agranulocytosis
- assess mental status prior to and during treatment
- monitor blood pressure
- ensure patient is taking medication
- monitor CBC and liver function tests
- instruct patient not to skip doses or double dose.

Cimetidine

Generic Name

cimetidine

Trade Name

Tagamet

Indication

treatment of duodenal ulcers, GERD, heartburn, Zollinger Ellison syndrome, prevention of GI bleeding in critical patients.

Action

inhibits action of histamine leading to inhibition of gastric acid secretion

Therapeutic Class

antiulcer agent

Pharmacologic Class

Histamine H2 antagonist

Nursing Considerations

- increases serum level of warfarin
- can lead to respiratory infection (green sputum)
- monitor for arryhtmias
- may cause agranulocytosis, aplastic anemia
- monitor CBC during therapy
- take medication as directed
- instruct patient to increase fluid and fiber intake to decrease constipation

Ciprofloxacin

Generic Name

ciprofloxacin

Trade Name

Cipro

Indication

urinary tract infections, gonorrhea, respiratory tract infections, bronchitis, pneumonia, skin and bone infections, infectious diarrhea, abdominal infections

Action

inhibits bacterial DNA synthesis

Therapeutic Class

anti-infectives

Pharmacologic Class

Fluoroquinolone

Nursing Considerations

- contraindicated in allergies
- may cause QT prolongation, avoid use with other drugs that can cause QT prolongation
- can cause seizures, arrythmias, pseudomembranous colitis, anaphalaxis, Stevens Johnson syndrome
- may decreased of phenytoin
- monitor renal panel
- assess for infection, obtain cultures prior to therapy
- monitor liver function tests

Clindamycin

Generic Name

clindamycin

Trade Name

Cleocin

Indication

skin infections, respiratory tract infections, septicemia, intra-abdominal infections, osteomyelitis

Action

inhibits protein synthesis

Therapeutic Class

Anti-infectives

Pharmacologic Class

none

Nursing Considerations

- arrythmias, pseudomembranous colitis, diarrhea, phlebitis
- monitor bowel function
- assess for infection, obtain cultures prior to therapy
- monitor liver function tests.
- monitor CBC

Clopidogrel

Generic Name

clopidogrel

Trade Name

Plavix

Indication

atherosclerotic events, MI, CVA, PVD, acute coronary syndrome

Action

inhibits platelet aggregation

Therapeutic Class

Antiplatelet agent

Pharmacologic Class

platelet aggregation inhibitors

Nursing Considerations

- may cause GI bleeding, neutropenia, hypercholesterolemia
- may increase risk for bleeding in warfarin, aspirin, heparin
- can increase risk for bleeding with garlic, ginkgo, ginger
- monitor for signs of bleeding
- monitor bleeding times
- monitor CBS and platelet count
- discontinue use 5-7 days before surgery

Codeine

Generic Name

codeine

Trade Name

Paveral

Indication

management of pain, diarrhea, cough suppressant

Action

Binds to opiate receptors in the CNS and alters perception of pain while producing a general depression of the CNS. This depression also causes a decrease in the cough reflex and GI motility.

Therapeutic Class

allergy, cold, cough remedy, antitussive, opioid analgesic

Pharmacologic Class

opioid agonist

Nursing Considerations

- may cause alterations in mentation, hypotension, constipation, nausea, vomiting
- assess BP, pulse, and respiratory rate prior to administration and frequently during administration
- use caution if patient is receiving MAO Inhibitors
- Narcan (naloxone) is the antidote for opioid agonists

Cortisone

Generic Name

cortisone

Trade Name

Cortone

Indication

management of adrenocortical insufficiency (Addison's Disease).

Action

Replace cortisol in states of deficiency, suppress inflammation and normal immune response. The adrenal glands sit on top of the kidneys. The adrenal glands excrete steroid hormones, including cortisol that play a role in increasing blood sugars, immune suppression, and metabolism of fat, protein, and carbohydrates, as well as decreasing bone formation.

Therapeutic Class

antiasthmatics, corticosteroids

Pharmacologic Class

corticosteroids

Nursing Considerations

- Excreted by the liver - monitor liver profile
- Avoid in active untreated infections
- may cause CNS alterations
- may cause peptic ulcers
- may cause Cushingoid appearance (buffalo hump, moon face)
- Weight gain
- Osteoporosis
- Decrease wound healing
- May elevate blood sugars

Cyclosporine

Generic Name

cyclosporine

Trade Name

Sandimmune

Indication

prevention of rejection in transplantation, treatment of severe RA, management of ulcerative colitis

Action

inhibits normal immune response

Therapeutic Class

immunosuppresants, antirheumatics (DMARD)

Pharmacologic Class

polypeptides (cyclic)

Nursing Considerations

- may cause seizures, tremors, hypertension, hepatotoxicity, diarrhea, N/V, gingival hyperplasia
- increases immune suppression with corticosteroids
- avoid grapefruit juice while taking this medications
- assess for signs of organ rejection
- monitor renal panel, liver enzymes
- take medication as directed
- lifelong therapy required for transplant patients
- instruct pt on how to take blood pressure

Dexamethasone

Generic Name

dexamethasone

Trade Name

Decadron

Indication

Manage cerebral edema, assess for Cushing's Disease

Action

Suppress inflammation and normal immune response. Used in inflammatory states to decrease inflammation.

Therapeutic Class

antiasthmatics, corticosteroids

Pharmacologic Class

corticosteroids

Nursing Considerations

- Excreted by the liver - monitor liver profile
- Avoid in active untreated infections
- may cause CNS alterations
- may cause peptic ulcers
- may cause Cushingoid appearance (buffalo hump, moon face)
- Weight gain
- Osteoporosis
- Decrease wound healing
- May elevate blood sugars
- May increase cholesterol and lipid values

Diazepam

Generic Name

diazepam

Trade Name

Valium

Indication
anxiety, pre-op sedation, conscious sedation, treatment of seizures, insomnia, management of alcohol withdrawal

Action

depresses the CNS

Therapeutic Class

antianxiety agents, anticonvulsants, sedative/hypnotics, skeletal muscle relaxants (centrally acting)

Pharmacologic Class

Benzodiazepine

Nursing Considerations

- contraindicated in hepatic dysfunction
- use caution with renal impairment
- can cause dizziness, drowsiness, lethargy, hypotension, physical dependence, tolerance
- instruct patient to take as directed
- caution to avoid alcohol use
- Romazicon is the reversal agent

Digoxin

Generic Name

digoxin

Trade Name

Lanoxin

Indication

CHF, A-fib, A-flutter

Action

Positive inotropic effect (increases force of myocardial contraction), prolongs refractory period, ↓ conduction through SA and AV nodes. Essentially digoxin is given to increase cardiac output and slow the rate.

Therapeutic Class

antiarrhythmic, inotropics

Pharmacologic Class

digitalis glycosides

Nursing Considerations

- Excreted by kidneys
- Assess patient for hypersensitivity
- Contraindicated with uncontrolled ventricular arryhtmias
- Hypokalemia increase risk for toxcicity
- Hypercalcemia ↑ risk for toxicity
- Use caution with diuretic use as they may cause electrolyte abnormalities that can lead to toxicity
- Assess patient for cardiac arrythmias including bradycardia
- Signs of toxicity include vision changes (blurred vision, yellow, green vision disturbances)

- Monitor pulse rate for 1 full minute prior to dosing patient (hold for pulse <60)

Diltiazem

Generic Name

diltiazem

Trade Name

Cardizem

Indication

hypertension, angina, SVT, a-fib, aflutter

Action

inhibits calcium transport resulting in inhibition of excitation and contraction, leads to vasodilatation and decreased blood pressure.

Therapeutic Class

antianginals, antiarrhythmics, antihypertensive

Pharmacologic Class

Ca Channel Blocker

Nursing Considerations

- contraindicated in 2nd and 3rd AV block
- may cause arryhtmias, CHF, bradycardia, peripheral edema, gingival hyperplasia
- increases digoxin levels
- don't drink grapefruit juice
- assess for signs of CHF
- monitor EKG continuously
- tell patient to change positions slowly

- monitor serum potassium
- instruct pt on how to take blood pressure

Diphenhydramine

Generic Name

diphenhydramine

Trade Name

Benadryl

Indication

allergy, anaphylaxis, sedation, motion sickness, antitussive

Action

antagonizes effects of histamine, CNS depression

Therapeutic Class

allergy, cold and cough remedy, antihistamine, antitussive

Pharmacologic Class

none

Nursing Considerations

- may cause drowsiness, anorexia, dry mouth, nausea, chest tightness, thick secretions, hypotension, blurred vision, headache
- anticholinergic effects
- assess purpose of medication prior to giving it
- assess allergies, sleep patters, cough and lung sounds
- patient should avoid other over-the-counter cough and cold remedies

Diphenoxylate/Atropine

Generic Name

diphenoxylate/atropine

Trade Name

Lomotil

Indication

Treatment for diarrhea

Action

Inhibits GI motility via anticholinergic effects

Therapeutic Class

antidiarrheal

Pharmacologic Class

anticholinergic

Nursing Considerations

- Contraindicated with angle-closure glaucoma, dehydration
- Structurally related to opioids so use caution with patients that have allergies to opioids
- Side effects: constipation, tachycardia, dizziness, ileus
- Monitor liver function as medication is excreted by the liver
- Insure that client is taking medication as prescribed and not double dosing

Divalproex

Generic Name

divalproex

Trade Name

Depakot

Indication

seizures, manic episodes, prevention of headache,
Action

increases the level of GABA in CNS

Therapeutic Class

Anticonvulsant, vascular headache suppressants

Pharmacologic Class

none

Nursing Considerations

- may cause suicidal thoughts, agitation, dizziness, insomnia, hepatotoxicity, pancreatitis
- increases risk for bleeding with Warfarin
- use caution with MAOIs
- monitor liver function tests

Dobutamine

Generic Name

dobutamine

Trade Name

Dobutrex

Indication

short term management of heart failure

Action

Dobutamine has a positive inotropic effect (increases cardiac output) with very little effect on heart rate. Stimulates Beta$_1$ receptors in the heart.

Therapeutic Class

inotropic

Pharmacologic Class

adrenergic

Nursing Considerations

- Monitor hemodynamics: hypertension, ↑HR, PVCs
- Skin reactions may occur with hypersensitivity
- Beta blockers may negate therapeutic effects of dobutamine
- Monitor cardiac output
- Monitor peripheral pulses before, during, and after therapy
- DO NOT confuse dobutamine with dopamine

Dopamine

Generic Name

dopamine

Trade Name

Intropin

Indication

used to improve blood pressure, cardiac output, and urine output

Action

Smaller doses result in renal vasodilation

Doses 2-10mcg/kg/min result in cardiac stimulation by acting on beta1 receptors

Doses >10mcg/kg/min stimulate alpha receptors leading to vasoconstriction (↑SVR)

Therapeutic Class

inotropic, vasopressor

Pharmacologic Class

adrenergic

Nursing Considerations

- Monitor hemodynamics closely: BP, HR, EKG, CVP, and PAOP if available
- Obtain parameters for hemodynamic values
- Titrate to obtain appropriate BP (more potent vasoconstrictors may be required)
- Irritation may occur at IV site

- Beta blockers may counteract therapeutic effects

Enalapril

Generic Name

enalopril

Trade Name

Vasotec

Indication
hypertension, management of CHF

Action

block conversion of angiotensin I to angiotensin II, increases renin levels and decreases aldosterone leading to vasodilation

Therapeutic Class

antihypertensives

Pharmacologic Class

ACE Inhibitor

Nursing Considerations

- can cause neutropenia - check WBCs regularly
- use cautiously with potassium supplements and potassium sparing diuretics.
- use cautiously with diuretic therapy
- administer 1 hour before meals
- monitor blood pressure often
- monitor weight and fluid status
- monitor renal profile
- monitor CBC frequently

Enoxaparin

Generic Name

enoxaparin

Trade Name

Lovenox

Indication

prevention of VTE, DVT, and PE

Action

prevents thrombus formation by potentiating the inhibitory effect of antithrombin on factor Xa and thrombin

Therapeutic Class

anticoagulant

Pharmacologic Class

antithrombotic

Nursing Considerations

- contraindicated in pork hypersensitivity
- monitor for signs of bleeding
- administer in subcutaneous tissue
- DO NOT eject air bubble prior to injection
- DO NOT aspirate or massage site

Epinephrine

Generic Name

epinephrine

Trade Name

Adrenalin, EpiPen

Indication

Asthma and COPD exacerbations, allergic reactions, cardiac arrest, anesthesia adjunct

Action

Affects both $beta_1$ and $beta_2$ also has alpha agonist properties. Results in bronchodilation, increases in HR and BP

Therapeutic Class

antiasthmatic, bronchodilator, vasopressor

Pharmacologic Class

adrenergic

Nursing Considerations

- Side effects include: angina, tachycardia, hypertension, restlessness, nervousness, hyperglycemia
- Use with MAOI may lead to hypertensive crisis
- Patients should not use stimulants (caffeine, guarana, etc)
- Excessive use may cause bronchospasm
- Assess lung sounds, pulse, BP, and other hemodynamic parameters
- Monitor for chest pain
- Instruct patient to use as directed
- Patient should insure adequate fluid intake to liquefy secretions
- Mouth should be rinsed after inhalation
- Beta blocker may negate effects

- May increase blood glucose levels

Epoetin

Generic Name

epoetin

Trade Name

Epogen

Indication

anemia

Action

stimulates erythropoesis

Therapeutic Class

antianemics

Pharmacologic Class

hormones

Nursing Considerations

- contraindicated in albumin hypersensitivity
- may cause seizures, CHF, MI, CVA, HTN
- monitor blood pressure during therapy
- monitor for signs of anemia
- assess dialysis shunts
- monitor bleeding times
- initiate seizure precautions
- do not shake vial

Erythromycin

Generic Name

erythromycin

Trade Name

E-Mycin

Indication

useful in place of penicillin when patient cannot take penicillin, upper and lower respiratory tract infections, otitis media, skin infections, pertussis, syphilis, rheumatic fever

Action

suppresses bacterial protein synthesis, bacteriostatic

Therapeutic Class

anti-infective

Pharmacologic Class

macrolide

Nursing Considerations

- Causes QT prolongation, ventricular arrhythmias
- diarrhea
- asses infection
- monitor liver function tests
- instruct patient to finish medication dosage even if they are feeling better
- medication should not be shared

Escitalopram

Generic Name

escitalopram

Trade Name

Lexapro

Indication

major depressive disorder, anxiety disorder, PCD, PTSD, social phobia

Action

selectively inhibits reuptake of serotonin

Therapeutic Class

Antidepressant

Pharmacologic Class

SSRI

Nursing Considerations

- contraindicated with MAOI and citallpran use
- may cause suicidal thoughts, insomnia, drowsiness, diarrhea, nausea, serotonin syndrome
- may cause QT prolongation with certain medications
- assess for sexual dysfunction
- may take 4-6 weeks for full affect to take place

Famotidine

Generic Name

famotidine

Trade Name

Pepcid

Indication

short term treatment of active ulcer, GERD, treatment of heartburn, indigestion, management of Zollinger Ellison syndrome, prevention of GI bleeding in critically ill patients, management of symptoms associated with overuse of NSAIDs

Action

blocks action of histamine located in gastric parietal cells, inhibits gastric acid secretion

Therapeutic Class

antiulcer agent

Pharmacologic Class

Histamine H2 antagonist

Nursing Considerations

- may cause arrythmias, agranulocytosis, aplastic anemias
- assess for abdominal pain and occult blood
- monitor CBC
- instruct pt to increase fluid and fiber intake to prevent constipation

Fentanyl

Generic Name

fentanyl

Trade Name

Sublimaze

Indication

supplement to general anesthesia, continuous IV infusion for purpose of analgesia

Action

binds to opiate receptors in CNS altering perception of pain, producing CNS depression

Therapeutic Class

Opioid Analgesic

Pharmacologic Class

opioid agonists

Nursing Considerations

- use caution with increased ICP, head trauma, adrenal insufficiency
- avoid use with MAOIs
- may cause apnea, laryngospasm, decreased respirations, bradycardia, hypotension
- do not consume grapefruit while taking this medication
- monitor hemodynamics during administration
- assess patient pain scale frequently

Ferrous sulfate

Generic Name

ferrous sulfate

Trade Name

Feosol

Indication

prevention and treatment of iron-deficiency anemia

Action

Iron is essential for hemoglobin, myoglobin and enzymes, it is transported to organs where it becomes part of iron stores

Therapeutic Class

antianemics

Pharmacologic Class

iron supplements

Nursing Considerations

- may cause seizures, hypotension, constipation, epigastric pain, diarrhea, skin staining, anaphylaxis
- assess nutritional status, bowel function
- monitor hemoglobin, hematocrit, iron levels
- may cause elevated liver enzymes
- take on an empty stomach to increase absorption/vitamin c helps with absorption
- use z-track for IM injections

Fluoxetine

Generic Name

fluoxetine

Trade Name

Prozac

Indication

depressive disorder, PCD, bulimia, panic disorder, bipolar, anorexia, ADHD, DM neuropathy, obesity

Action

inhibits reuptake of serotonin

Therapeutic Class

Antidepressant

Pharmacologic Class

SSRI

Nursing Considerations

- do not use while taking MAOIs
- may cause suicidal thoughts, drowsiness, anxiety, sexual dysfunction, insomnia, palpitations
- monitor closely for serotonin syndrome
- concurrent use with certain medications may lead to QT prolongation
- monitor mood changes and assess for suicidal ideation
- monitor nutrition status
- may cause elevated liver enzymes
- instruct pt to maintain good oral hygiene

Fluticasone

Generic Name

Fluticasone

Trade Name

Flovent

Indication

prophylactic asthma treatment

Action

locally acting anti-inflammatory

Therapeutic Class

antiasthmatics, anti-inflammatory (steroid)

Pharmacologic Class

Coticosteroids, Inhalation

Nursing Considerations

- use cautiously with untreated infections and suppressed immune function
- may cause headache, insomnia, bronchospasm, nasal congestion, adrenal suppression
- monitor patient's respiratory status
- may lead to decreased bone density
- instruct patients using corticosteroids and bronchodilators that they need to use bronchodilators first.
- instruct patient to stop smoking

Furosemide

Generic Name

Furosemide

Trade Name

Lasix

Indication

edema, hypertension

Action

prevents reabsorption of sodium and chloride in the kidneys, increase excretion of water, sodium, chloride, magnesium, potassium.

Therapeutic Class

Diuretics

Pharmacologic Class

loop diuretics

Nursing Considerations

- use caution with liver disease
- may cause hypotension, dry mouth, excessive urination, dehydration, electrolyte abnormalities, metabolic alkalosis
- hypokalemia may lead to increase risk of digoxin toxicity
- monitor renal panel
- use caution with other anithypertensives
- causes arthritic symptoms/do not administer with aminoglycosides due to ototoxicity

Gabapentine

Generic Name

gabapentine

Trade Name

Neurontin

Indication

seizures, peripheral neuropathy, neuropathic pain, prevention of migraines

Action

exact method of action unknown

Therapeutic Class

analgesic adjuncts, therapeutic, anticonvulsants, mood stabilizers

Pharmacologic Class

none

Nursing Considerations

- may cause suicidal thoughts, confusion, depression, drowsiness, ataxia, facial edema, hypertension
- monitor pt closely for changes in behavior and depression
- assess seizure activity
- assess pain level
- patient should take medications exactly as prescribed

Gentamicin

Generic Name

gentamicin

Trade Name

cidomycin

Indication

Treatment of gram negative infections when penicillin is ineffective

Action

Inhibits bacterial protein synthesis

Therapeutic Class

anti-infectives

Pharmacologic Class

Aminoglycoside

Nursing Considerations

- causes tinnitus-hearing loss/do not administer with penicillin
- use caution in renal impairment
- assess for infection
- obtain cultures prior to therapy
- monitor liver function tests
- monitor blood levels of drug

Glipizide

Generic Name

glipizide

Trade Name

Glucotrol

Indication

type 2 diabetes mellitus

Action

stimulates release and sensitivity to insulin to lower blood glucose

Therapeutic Class

anti-diabetic

Pharmacologic Class

sulfonylureas

Nursing Considerations

- may cause aplastic anemias, hypoglycemia, photosensitivity, dizziness, drowsiness, headache, diarrhea
- monitor CBC, assess for allergy to sulfonamides
- beta blockers may create signs of hypoglycemia
- instruct patient on how to check blood sugars and
- instruct patient on importance of carrying source of sugar in case of hypoglycemia

Glucagon

Generic Name

glucagon

Trade Name

GlucaGen

Indication

Severe hypoglycemia, antidote for Beta Blockers and calcium channel blockers

Action

Stimulates production of glucose, relaxes Gi tract,

Therapeutic Class

hormones

Pharmacologic Class

pancreatics

Nursing Considerations

- may cause anaphylaxis
- may cause hypotension
- assess for signs of hypoglycemia, neuro status
- monitor serum glucose levels
- teach patient signs of hypoglycemia

Guaifenesin

Generic Name

Guaifenesin

Trade Name

Robitussin

Indication

Cough suppression

Action

Decreases viscosity of and mobilizes secretions

Therapeutic Class

allergy, cold and cough remedies, expectorant

Pharmacologic Class

none

Nursing Considerations

- patient should avoid over the counter cold medications
- assess lung sounds
- maintain adequate fluid intake

Haloperidol

Generic Name

haloperidol

Trade Name

Haldol

Indication

Schizophrenia, mania, aggressive and agitated patient

Action

Alters the effect of dopamine

Therapeutic Class

Antipsychotic

Pharmacologic Class

butyrophenones

Nursing Considerations

- extrapyramidal symptoms

- use caution in QT prolongation
- may cause seizures, constipation, dry mouth, agranulosytosis
- assess for hallucinations
- monitor hemodynamics
- monitor for neuroleptic malignant syndrome
- monitor CBC with differential

Heparin

Generic Name

heparin

Trade Name

Hep-Lock

Indication

Venous thromboembolism prophylaxis and treatment, low dose used to ensure patency of IV catheters

Action

increases the inhibitory effect of antithrombin on factor Xa

Therapeutic Class

anticoagulant

Pharmacologic Class

antithrombotic

Nursing Considerations

- monitor for signs of bleeding
- monitor platelet count
- may cause hyperkalemia
- have patient report any signs of bleeding

Hydralazine

Generic Name

hydralazine

Trade Name

Apresoline

Indication

hypertension

Action

arterial vasodilator

Therapeutic Class

anti-hypertensive

Pharmacologic Class

vasodilator

Nursing Considerations

- may cause tachycardia, sodium retention, arrhythmias, angina
- use caution with MAOIs
- monitor blood pressure
- instruct patient on how to take blood pressure

Hydrochlorothiazide

Generic Name

hydrochlorothiazide

Trade Name

Hydrodiuril

Indication

Hypertension, CHF, renal dysfunction, cirrhosis, glucocorticoid therapy

Action

Increases sodium and water excretion produces arteriol dilation

Therapeutic Class

antihypertensives, diuretics

Pharmacologic Class

thiazide diuretics

Nursing Considerations

- May cause dizziness, hypokalemia, hyponatremia, hypophosphatemia, hypomadnesemia, dehydration
- Hypokalemia can increase risk for digoxin toxicity
- Monitor blood pressure and intake and output
- Monitor electrolyte levels
- Patient should take medication at the same time each day even if feeling better
- Instruct patient on how to take blood pressure

Hydrocodone/Acetaminophen

Generic Name

hydrocodone/acetaminophen

Trade Name

Norco

Indication

management of moderate to severe pain

Action

alters the perception and reaction to pain by binding to opiate receptors in the CNS, also suppresses the cough reflex

Therapeutic Class

opioid Analgesic, allergy, cold and cough remedies, antitussive

Pharmacologic Class

opioid agonists, nonopioid analgesic combinations

Nursing Considerations

- use caution with concurrent use of MAOI - avoid use within 14 days of each other
- hypotension - monitor hemodynamics and respirations after administering
- may increase ICP use caution with head trauma
- Narcan is the antidote for overdose
- do not exceed 4g of acetaminophen per day

Hydromorphone

Generic Name

hydromorphone

Trade Name

Dilaudid

Indication

moderate to severe pain

Action

alters the perception and reaction to pain by binding to opiate receptors in the CNS, also suppresses the cough reflex

Therapeutic Class

Opioid Analgesic, allergy, cold and cough remedies, antitussive

Pharmacologic Class

opioid agonist

Nursing Considerations

- Assess BP, respirations, and pulse before and during administration - medication causes general CNS depression
- Narcan is the antidote for overdose
- use caution with concurrent use of MAOI - avoid use within 14 days of each other
- may be used as an antitussive
- advised to dilute with NS prior to administration and to administer slowly to decrease CNS depression

Ibuprofen

Generic Name

ibuprofen

Trade Name

Advil / Motrin

Indication

Mild to moderate pain, inflammatory states

Action

Decreases pain and inflammation by inhibiting prostaglandins

Therapeutic Class

antipyretics, antirheumatics, nonopioid analgesics, nonsteroidal anti-inflammatory agents

Pharmacologic Class

nonopioid analgesics

Nursing Considerations

- may cause GI bleeding, hepatitis, Stevens-Johnson Syndrome
- may cause anaphylaxis
- monitor for headache, nausea, vomiting, constipation
- therapy should be discontinued after first sign of rash
- monitor renal and liver labs
- patient should avoid using alcohol

Indomethacin

Generic Name

indomethacin

Trade Name

Indocin

Indication

Inflammatory disorders when patients do not respond to other medications

Action

Decreases pain and inflammation by inhibiting prostaglandin synthesis

Therapeutic Class

antirheumatics, ductus arteriosus patency adjuncts (IV only), nonsteroidal anti-inflammatory agents

Pharmacologic Class

none

Nursing Considerations

- Monitor for hepatitis and GI bleeding
- Monitor for dizziness, drowsiness, and headache
- Assess for anaphylactic reaction
- Aspirin may decrease effectiveness
- Monitor renal labs
- Shake suspension before administration
- Patient should wear sunscreen and protective clothing to protect against photosensitivity

Insulin- short acting

Generic Name

regular

Trade Name

Humulin R/Novolin R

Indication

hyperglycemia with diabetes type 1 and 2, diabetic ketoacidosis

Action

stimulates uptake of glucose into muscle and fat cells, inhibits production of glucose in the liver, prevents breakdown of fat and protein

Route	Onset	Peak	Duration
IV	1-2 hr	4-12 hr	18-24

Therapeutic Class

antidiabetics, hormones

Pharmacologic Class

pancreatics

Nursing Considerations

- assess for symptoms of hypoglycemia or hyperglycemia
- monitor body weight over time
- may cause decreased inorganic phosphates, potassium, and magnesium
- monitor blood sugars every 6 hours, monitor A1C every 3-6 months

Insulin- intermediate acting

Generic Name

NPH

Trade Name

Humulin N, Novolin N

Indication

hyperglycemia with diabetes type 1 and 2, diabetic ketoacidosis

Action

stimulates uptake of glucose into muscle and fat cells, inhibits production of glucose in the liver, prevents breakdown of fat and protein

Route	Onset	Peak	Duration
IV	10-30 min	15-30 min	30-60 min
Subcutaneous	30-60 min	2-4 hr	5-7 hr

Therapeutic Class

antidiabetics, hormones

Pharmacologic Class

pancreatics

Nursing Considerations

- assess for symptoms of hypoglycemia or hyperglycemia
- monitor body weight over time
- may cause decreased inorganic phosphates, potassium, and magnesium
- monitor blood sugars every 6 hours, monitor A1C every 3-6 months

Insulin- long acting

Generic Name

detemir, glargine

Trade Name

Levemir, Lantus

Indication

hyperglycemia with diabetes type 1 and 2, diabetic ketoacidosis

Action

stimulates uptake of glucose into muscle and fat cells, inhibits production of glucose in the liver, prevents breakdown of fat and protein

Route	Onset	Peak	Duration
Detemir	3-4 hr	3-14 hr	24 hr
Glargine	3-4 hr	none	24 hr

Therapeutic Class

antidiabetics, hormones

Pharmacologic Class

pancreatics

Nursing Considerations

- assess for symptoms of hypoglycemia or hyperglycemia
- monitor body weight over time
- may cause decreased inorganic phosphates, potassium, and magnesium
- monitor blood sugars every 6 hours, monitor A1C every 3-6 months

Insulin- rapid acting

Generic Name

aspart, lispro, glulisine

Trade Name

novolog, humalog, apidra

Indication

hyperglycemia with diabetes type 1 and 2, diabetic ketoacidosis

Action

stimulates uptake of glucose into muscle and fat cells, inhibits production of glucose in the liver, prevents breakdown of fat and protein

Route	Onset	Peak	Duration
Aspart	10-20 min	1-3 hr	3-5 hr
Glulisine	15 min	1 hr	2-4 hr
Lispro	15 min	1-1.5 hr	3-4 hr

Therapeutic Class

antidiabetics, hormones

Pharmacologic Class

pancreatics

Nursing Considerations

- assess for symptoms of hypoglycemia or hyperglycemia
- monitor body weight over time
- may cause decreased inorganic phosphates, potassium, and magnesium
- monitor blood sugars every 6 hours, monitor A1C every 3-6 months

Insulin-mixtures

Generic Name

Lispro mixture, Aspart mixture, NPH/regular

Trade Name

Humalog Mix, NovoLog Mix, Humulin 70/30, Novolin 70/30

Indication

hyperglycemia with diabetes type 1 and 2, diabetic ketoacidosis

Action

stimulates uptake of glucose into muscle and fat cells, inhibits production of glucose in the liver, prevents breakdown of fat and protein

Route	Onset	Peak	Duration
Lispro mix	15-30 min	2-3 hr	24 hr
Aspart mix	15 min	1-4 hr	18-24 hr
NPH regular	30 min	4-8 hr	24 hr

Therapeutic Class

antidiabetics, hormones

Pharmacologic Class

pancreatics

Nursing Considerations

- assess for symptoms of hypoglycemia or hyperglycemia
- monitor body weight over time
- may cause decreased inorganic phosphates, potassium, and magnesium
- monitor blood sugars every 6 hours, monitor A1C every 3-6 months

Iodine

Generic Name

radioactive iodine

Trade Name

none

Indication

thyroidectomy, thyrotoxic crisis, radiation exposure

Action

inhibits the release of thyroid hormones

Therapeutic Class

Antithyroid Agent

Pharmacologic Class

none

Nursing Considerations

- may cause GI bleeding, diarrhea, hypothyroidism, goiter
- monitor for hypersensitivity

Isoniazide

Generic Name

isoniazide

Trade Name

INH

Indication

tuberculosis

Action

Inhibits synthesis of mycobacterial cell wall

Therapeutic Class

Antitubercular

Pharmacologic Class

none

Nursing Considerations

- can cause jaundice
- may cause peripheral neuropathy, seizures, hepatitis
- patient should avoid high amounts of tyramine
- monitor liver function tests

Ketorolac

Generic Name

ketorolac

Trade Name

Toradol

Indication

pain

Action

Pain relief due to prostaglandin inhibition

Therapeutic Class

nonsteroidal anti-inflammatory agents, nonopioid analgesics

Pharmacologic Class

pyrroziline carboxylic acid

Nursing Considerations

- may cause GI bleeding, Stevens-Johnson Syndrome, anaphylaxis, drowsiness
- should not exceed 5 days of therapy
- bleeding risk increased with garlic, ginger, and ginkgo
- may decrease effectiveness of hypertensive medications and diuretics

Lactulose

Generic Name

lactulose

Trade Name

Kristalose

Indication

Constipation, portal-systemic encephalopathy

Action

Draws water into the stool and softens stool, inhibits ammonia passing into the colon

Therapeutic Class

laxative

Pharmacologic Class

osmotic

Nursing Considerations

- use caution with DM
- may cause cramps, abdominal distention, hyperglycemia
- assess mental status, ammonia levels, abdominal distention
- patient should average 2-3 bowel movements per day

Lamotrigine

Generic Name

lamotrigine

Trade Name

Lamictal

Indication

Seizures r/t epilepsy, bipolar

Action

Inhibits sodium transport in neurons

Therapeutic Class

anticonvulsant

Nursing Considerations

- May cause suicidal thoughts, dizziness, behavior changes, nausea, vomiting, photosensitivity, rash, Stevens-Johnson Syndrome
- Use caution with oral contraceptive use
- Assess mental status
- Assess for seizures
- Do not discontinue use abruptly

Levetiracetam

Generic Name

levetiracetam

Trade Name

Keppra

Indication

Seizures

Action

Decreases severity and incidence of seizures

Therapeutic Class

anticonvulsants

Pharmacologic Class

pyrrolidines

Nursing Considerations

- May cause suicidal thoughts, dizziness, weakness
- May alter RBC, WBC, and liver function
- May cause somnolence
- Should be infused over 15 minutes

Levofloxacin

Generic Name

levofloxacin

Trade Name

Levaquin

Indication

urinary tract infections, gonorrhea, respiratory tract infections, bronchitis, pneumonia, skin and bone infections

Action

Inhibits DNA synthesis in bacteria

Therapeutic Class

Anti-infective

Pharmacologic Class

fluoroquinolone

Nursing Considerations

- contraindicated in allergies
- may cause QT prolongation, avoid use with other drugs that can cause QT prolongation
- can cause seizures, arrythmias, pseudomembranous colitis, anaphylaxis, Stevens Johnson syndrome
- may decreased of phenytoin
- monitor renal panel
- assess for infection, obtain cultures prior to therapy
- monitor liver function tests

Levothyroxine

Generic Name

levothyroxine

Trade Name

Levothroid

Indication

thyroid hormone replacement in hypothyroidism

Action

replaces thyroid hormone increasing metabolism, promotes gluconeogenesis, stimulates protein synthesis, restores normal hormone balance and suppresses thyroid cancer

Therapeutic Class

hormone

Pharmacologic Class

thyroid preparations

Nursing Considerations

- assess pulse and monitor for tachyarrythmias and chest pain
- monitor TSH levels
- overdose is presented as hyperthyroidism
- start with low doses and increase as indicated
- therapy is lifelong
- take directly after breast feeding
- increases the effects of warfarin

Lisipnorpil

Generic Name

lisinopril

Trade Name

Prinivil

Indication

hypertension, management of CHF

Action

block conversion of angiotensin I to angiotensin II, increases renin levels and decreases aldosterone leading to vasodilation

Therapeutic Class

antihypertensives

Pharmacologic Class

ACE Inhibitor

Nursing Considerations

- use cautiously with potassium supplements and potassium sparing diuretics.
- use cautiously with diuretic therapy
- administer 1 hour before meals
- monitor blood pressure often
- monitor weight and fluid status
- monitor renal profile
- monitor liver function tests

Lithium

Generic Name

lithium

Trade Name

Lithizine

Indication

mania

Action

alters cation transport and neurotransmitter reuptake

Therapeutic Class

Mood Stabilizer

Pharmacologic Class

none

Nursing Considerations

- do not administer with NSAIDs
- monitor drug blood levels frequently
- may cause seizures arrhythmia, EKG changes, fatigue, confusion, nausea, anorexia, hypothyroidisms, tremors
- Ace Inhibitors may increase serum levels
- instruct patient to maintain adequate fluid intake
- therapeutic level: 0.5-1.5 mEq/L

Loperamide

Generic Name

loperamide

Trade Name

Imodium

Indication

acute diarrhea, decrease drainage post ileostomy

Action

inhibits peristalsis, reduces the volume of feces while increasing the bulk and viscosity

Therapeutic Class

antidiarrheal

Nursing Considerations

- may lead to constipation - insure proper use
- assess bowel function
- assess fluid and electrolyte levels

Loarazepam

Generic Name

lorazepam

Trade Name

Ativan

Indication

anxiety, sedation

Action

general CNS depression

Therapeutic Class

anesthetic adjuncts, antianxiety agents, sedative hypnotics

Pharmacologic Class

Benzodiazepine

Nursing Considerations

- use caution with COPD and sleep apnea
- avoid alcohol use
- antidote is Flumazenil
- may cause apnea, cardiac arrest, bradycardia, hypotension
- use caution with other CNS depressants
- administer slowly and dilute to decrease complications

Losartan

Generic Name

Losartan

Trade Name

Cozaar

Indication

hypertension, DM neuropathy, CHF

Action

inhibits vasoconstrictive properties of angiotensin II

Therapeutic Class

antihypertensives

Pharmacologic Class

angiotensin II receptor antagonist

Nursing Considerations

- may cause hypotension, tacycardia, angiodema, hyperkalemia,
- may increase digoxin levels
- assess blood pressure and heart rate
- assess fluid levels
- monitor daily weights with CHF
- monitor renal and liver
- instruct patient on how to take blood pressure

Magnesium sulfate

Generic Name

magnesium sulfate

Trade Name

MgSO4

Indication

treatment of hypomagnesaemia, hypertension, preterm labor, torsade de pointes, asthma, anticonvulsant with eclampsia

Action

magnesium plays a role in muscle excitability

Therapeutic Class

mineral and electrolyte replacements/supplements

Pharmacologic Class

minerals/electrolytes

Nursing Considerations

- use caution with renal insufficiency
- may cause decreased respiratory rate, arrythmias, hypotension, muscle weakness
- monitor EKG and respiratory status
- monitor Mg levels
- ensure dosage with secondary practitioner

Mannitol

Generic Name

mannitol

Trade Name

Osmitrol

Indication

increased ICP, oliguric renal failure, edema, intraocular pressure

Action

inhibits reabsorptions of water and electrolytes by increasing osmotic pressure, excreted by kidneys

Therapeutic Class

Pharmacologic Class

Nursing Considerations

- may cause phlebitis at IV site
- may cause dehydration, fluid and electrolyte imbalances
- monitor neuro status

Methylprednisone

Generic Name

methylprednisone

Trade Name

Solu-medrol

Indication

Inflammation, allergy, autoimmune disorders, prevent organ rejection

Action

suppress inflammation and normal immune response, the adrenal glands sit on top of the kidneys. The adrenal glands excrete steroid hormones that play a role in increasing blood sugars, immune suppression, and metabolism of fat, protein, and carbohydrates, as well as decreasing bone formation.

Therapeutic Class

antiasthmatics, corticosteroids

Pharmacologic Class

corticosteroids

Nursing Considerations

- Excreted by the liver - monitor liver profile
- Avoid in active untreated infections
- may cause CNS alterations
- may cause peptic ulcers
- may cause Cushingoid appearance (buffalo hump, moon face)
- Weight gain
- Osteoporosis
- Decrease wound healing
- May elevate blood sugars
- May increase cholesterol and lipid values

- depress immune system/report signs of infection (soar throat)
- avoid grapefruit juice

Meperidine

Generic Name

meperidine

Trade Name

Demerol

Indication

moderate to severe pain, sedation

Action

Binds to opiate receptors in the CNS and alters perception of pain while producing a general depression of the CNS.

Therapeutic Class

Opioid Analgesic

Pharmacologic Class

opioid agonists

Nursing Considerations

- may cause alterations in mentation, hypotension, constipation, nausea, vomiting
- assess BP, pulse, and respiratory rate prior to administration and frequently during administration
- use caution if patient is receiving MAOIs
- Narcan (naloxone) is the antidote for opioid agonists
- can cause seizure
- may increase pancreatic enzyme levels

- assess bowel function

Metformin

Generic Name

metformin

Trade Name

Glucophage

Indication

management of Type II DM

Action

decreases glucose production in the liver, decreases absorption, increases cellular insulin sensitivity.

Therapeutic Class

Antidiabetic

Pharmacologic Class

Biguanide

Nursing Considerations

- do not use with renal dysfunction, metabolic acidosis
- may cause diarrhea, nausea, vomiting, lactic acidosis
- monitor patient closely for ketoacidosis and lactic acidosis, discontinue medication immediately if acidotic
- may cause metallic taste
- instruct patient that medication does not cure diabetes

Methadone

Generic Name

methadone

Trade Name

Mathadose

Indication

withdrawal symptoms, pain

Action

Binds to opiate receptors in the CNS and alters perception of pain while producing a general depression of the CNS. This depression also causes a decrease in the cough reflex and GI motility.

Therapeutic Class

opioid analgesic

Pharmacologic Class

opioid agonist

Nursing Considerations

- use caution if patient is receiving MAO Inhibitors
- may cause QT prolongation, hypotension, respiratory depression, dependence, confusion, sedation
- assess pain, vital signs, bowel function
- may increase pancreatic enzyme levels
- assess withdrawal symptoms

Methylergonovine

Generic Name

methylergonovine

Trade Name

Methergine

Indication

treatment of post-partum hemorrhage

Action

stimulates uterine muscles causing uterine contraction

Therapeutic Class

oxytocic

Pharmacologic Class

ergot alkaloids

Nursing Considerations

- can cause hypertension, cramps, nausea, vomiting, dyspnea
- monitor BP, heart rate, uterine response
- assess calcium levels

Methylphenidate

Generic Name

methylphenidate

Trade Name

Ritalin

Indication

ADHD, narcolepsy

Action

improves attention span in ADHD by producing CNS stimulation

Therapeutic Class

central nervous system stimulant

Pharmacologic Class

none

Nursing Considerations

- can cause sudden death, hypertension, palpitations, anorexia, hyperactivity, insomnia
- may decrease effects of Warfarin and Phenytoin
- do not use with MAOIs
- monitor cardiovascular system
- monitor for behavioral changes
- monitor for dependence
- do not consume caffeinated beverages

Metoclopramide

Generic Name

metoclopramide

Trade Name

Reglan

Indication

prevention of nausea, vomiting, hiccups, migraines, gastric stasis

Action

accelerates gastric emptying by stimulating motility

Therapeutic Class

antiemetic

Pharmacologic Class

none

Nursing Considerations

- don't use with GI obstruction
- may cause extrapyramidal reaction, neurolyptic malignant syndrome, tardive dyskinesia, arrhythmias, blood pressure alterations, hematologic alterations, facial movements, sedation
- can decrease effects of levodopa
- assess nausea/vomiting
- monitor liver function tests

Metoprolol

Generic Name

metoprolol

Trade Name

Lopressor

Indication

HTN, angina, prevention of MI, heart failure management, may be used for migraine prophylaxis

Action

blocks the stimulation of $beta_1$ receptors in the SNS with does not usually effect on $beta_2$ receptors (cardioselective)

Therapeutic Class

antianginal, antihypertensive

Pharmacologic Class

beta blocker

Nursing Considerations

- monitor hemodynamics
- may lead to bradycardia, pulmonary edema
- use caution with MAOIs
- assess I&Os and monitor for signs of CHF

Metronidazole

Generic Name

metronidazole

Trade Name

Flagyl

Indication

intra-abdominal infections, gynecoligical infections, skin infections, bone and joint infections, CNS infections, septicemia, endocarditis, amebic liver abscess, peptic ulcer disease,

Action

Inhibits DNA and protein synthesis in bacteria, bactericidal

Therapeutic Class

anti-infectives, antiprotozoals, antiulcer agents

Pharmacologic Class

none

Nursing Considerations

- do not take with alcohol-disulfiram reaction
- assess for infection before and during treatment
- obtain cultures before therapy
- monitor neurologic status: parasthesia, weakness, ataxia, or seizures
- monitor intake and output, daily weights
- may alter liver enzyme tests

Midazolam

Generic Name

midazolam

Trade Name

Versed

Indication

sedation, conscious sedation, anesthesia, status epilepticus

Action

Acts to produce CNS depression, may be mediated by GABA.

Therapeutic Class

Antianxiety agent, sedative/hypnotics

Pharmacologic Class

Benzodiazepine

Nursing Considerations

- assess level of sedation during and for 2-6 hours following
- monitor blood pressure, pulse, respirations during IV administration
- The antidote for overdose is flumazenil

Montelukast

Generic Name

montelukast

Trade Name

Singulair

Indication

prevent or treat asthma, manage seasonal allergies, prevent exercise-induced bronchoconstriction

Action

disrupts the effects of leukotrienes which effect ariway edema, smooth muscle constriction, and cellular activity.

Therapeutic Class

allergy, cold, and cough remedies, bronchodilators

Pharmacologic Class

Leukotriene Antagonist

Nursing Considerations

- assess respiratory status
- assess liver function tests
- medication does not treat acute asthma attacks

Morphine

Generic Name

morphine

Trade Name

MS Contin

Indication

pain, pulmonary edema, MI

Action

Binds to opiate receptors in the CNS and alters perception of pain while producing a general depression of the CNS. This depression also causes a decrease in the cough reflex and GI motility.

Therapeutic Class

opioid analgesic

Pharmacologic Class

opioid agonist

Nursing Considerations

- may cause alterations in mentation, hypotension, constipation, nausea, vomiting
- assess BP, pulse, and respiratory rate prior to administration and frequently during administration
- use caution if patient is receiving MAO Inhibitors
- Narcan (naloxone) is the antidote for opioid agonists

Nalbuphine

Generic Name

nalbuphine

Trade Name

Nubain

Indication

pain, analgesia during labor, sedation before surgery, supplement to balance anesthesia

Action

alters perception and response to pain, causes CNS depression

Therapeutic Class

Opioid Analgesic

Pharmacologic Class

opioid agonists/analgesics

Nursing Considerations

- use caution with head trauma
- can cause dizziness, headache, nausea, vomiting, respiratory depression
- do not use with MAOIs
- assess pain
- asses hemodynamic parameters
- may elevate pancreatic enzymes
- narcan is the antidote

Naproxen

Generic Name

naproxen

Trade Name

Aleve

Indication

pain, dismenorrhea, fever, inflammation

Action

inhibits prostaglandin

Therapeutic Class

nonsteroidal anti-inflammatory agents, nonopioid analgesics, antipyretics

Pharmacologic Class

none

Nursing Considerations

- use caution with GI bleeding
- may increase risk for stroke and MI
- can cause GI bleeding, anaphylaxis, Steven's Johnson syndrome
- aspirin can decrease blood levels and effectiveness
- assess pain
- patients should remain up-right for 30 minutes after administration

Nifedipine

Generic Name

nifedipine

Trade Name

Procardia

Indication

hypertension, angina, migraines, CHF

Action

blocks calcium transport resulting in inhibition of contraction causing systemic vasodilatation

Therapeutic Class

antianginals, antihypertensives

Pharmacologic Class

Ca Channel Blocker

Nursing Considerations

- use caution in heart block, decreased blood pressure
- don't consume grapefruit juice while taking medication
- may cause arrhythmias
- may cause elevated liver function tests
- may cause gingival hyperplasia, Steven's Johnson syndrome
- monitor blood pressure and pulse
- monitor calcium levels
- instruct patient on taking heart rate and blood pressure

Nitroprusside

Generic Name

nitroprusside

Trade Name

Nitropress

Indication

hypertensive crisis, cardiogenic shock

Action

peripheral vasodilation of arteries and veins decreasing preload and afterload

Therapeutic Class

antihypertensive

Pharmacologic Class

vasodilator

Nursing Considerations

- monitor HR, BP, and EKG continuously during therapy
- may cause cyanide toxicity
- sympathomimetics may decrease effectiveness
- PAOP monitoring may help with MI and CHF patients

Norepnephrine

Generic Name

norepinephrine

Trade Name

Levophed

Indication

treatment of severe hypotension and shock

Action

increase blood pressure and cardiac output by stimulating alpha-adrenergic receptors in the blood vessels, demonstrates minor beta activity

Therapeutic Class

vasopressor

Nursing Considerations

- monitor BP continuously if possible or every couple of minutes
- double check all concentrations with additional nurse
- may result in rebound hypotension due to tissue ischemia when discontinued
- monitor EKG and CVP if possible
- if patient is awake instruct them to report headaches, dizziness, or chest pain

Nystatin

Generic Name

nystatin

Trade Name

Mycostatin

Indication

candidiasis

Action

causes leakage of fungal cell contents

Therapeutic Class

Antifungal

Pharmacologic Class

none

Nursing Considerations

- may cause diarrhea, nausea, vomiting
- use caution with dentures
- assess mucus membrane

Olanzapine

Generic Name

olanzapine

Trade Name

Zyprexa

Indication

schizophrenia, mania, depression, anorexia nervosa, nausea/vomiting related to chemotherapy

Action

antagonizes dopamine and serotonin

Therapeutic Class

Antipsychotic, mood stabilizers

Pharmacologic Class

thienobenzodiazeoines

Nursing Considerations

- do not use while breastfeeding
- can cause neurolyptic malignant syndrome, seizures, suicidal thoughts, insomnia, tardive dyskinesia, aggranulocytosis, constipation, tremors
- assess mental status
- monitor hemodynamics
- assess blood sugars
- assess intake and output
- monitor liver function tests

Omeprazole

Generic Name

omeprazole

Trade Name

Prilosec

Indication

GERD, ulcers, Zollinger-Ellison syndrome, reduce the risk of GI bleed in critically ill patients, heart burn

Action

prevents the transport of H ions into the gastric lumen by binding to gastric parietal cells

Therapeutic Class

antiulcer agent

Pharmacologic Class

proton-pump inhibitor

Nursing Considerations

- capsules should be swallowed whole
- instruct patient to report black tarry stool

Ondansetron

Generic Name

ondansetron

Trade Name

Zofran

Indication

nausea/vomiting

Action

blocks effects of serotonin on vagal nerve and CNS

Therapeutic Class

Antiemetic

Pharmacologic Class

5-HT3 antagonist

Nursing Considerations

- may cause headache, constipation, diarrhea, dry mouth
- asses nausea and vomiting
- assess for extrapyramidal symptoms
- monitor liver function tests
- administer slowly over 2-5 minutes

Oxycodone

Generic Name

oxycodone

Trade Name

Oxycontin

Indication

pain

Action

binds to opiate receptors in CNS

Therapeutic Class

Opioid Analgesic

Pharmacologic Class

opioid agonists, opioid agonists/nonopioid, analgesic combinations

Nursing Considerations

- may cause respiratory depression, constipation, confusion , sedation, hallucinations, urinary retention
- use caution with increased intracranial pressure
- don't use with MAOIs
- assess hemodynamics
- assess pain
- may elevate pancreatic enzymes
- can cause physical dependence
- assess bowel function

Oxytocin

Generic Name

oxytocin

Trade Name

Pitocin

Indication

labor induction, postpartum bleeding

Action

stimulates uterine smooth muscle

Therapeutic Class

hormones

Pharmacologic Class

oxytocics

Nursing Considerations

- can cause ICH in fetus
- can cause asphyxia in fetus
- may cause coma and seizures in mother
- may cause painful contractions
- assess fetus
- assess contractions
- monitor blood pressure
- assess maternal electrolytes
- may cause uterine tetany

Pancrealipase

Generic Name

pancrelipase

Trade Name

Creon

Indication

pancreatic insufficiency, ductal obstruction

Action

replacement of pancreatic enzymes: lipase, amylase, protease

Therapeutic Class

digestive agent

Pharmacologic Class

pancreatic enzyme

Nursing Considerations

- contraindicated with pig products
- can cause shortness of breath, nausea, diarrhea, rash
- assess nutritional status
- monitor for steatorrhea
- may increase uric acid levels
- instruct patient to follow diet
- take with meals and snacks

Pantoprazole

Generic Name

pantoprazole

Trade Name

Protonix

Indication

GERD, heartburn

Action

decreases accumulation of acid in the stomach

Therapeutic Class

antiulcer agents

Pharmacologic Class

proton-pump inhibitors

Nursing Considerations

- can cause hyperglycemia, abdominal pain
- decreases absorption of certain drugs
- may increase bleeding with warfarin
- assess for occult blood
- assess liver enzymes

Paroxetine

Generic Name

paroxetine

Trade Name

Paxil

Indication

major depressive disorder, OCD, anxiety, PTSD

Action

block reuptake of serotonin in CNS

Therapeutic Class

antianxiety agent, antidepressant

Pharmacologic Class

SSRI

Nursing Considerations

- do not use with MAOIs
- can cause neurolyptic malignant syndrome, suicidal thoughts, serotonin syndrome, constipation, diarrhea, insomnia
- decrease effectiveness of digoxin
- increase bleeding with warfarin
- assess for suicidal thoughts

Phenazopyridine

Generic Name

phenazopyridine

Trade Name

Pyridium

Indication

urological pain

Action

provides analgesia to the urinary tract mucosa

Therapeutic Class

nonopioid analgesics

Pharmacologic Class

urinary tract analgesics

Nursing Considerations

- will turn urine red or orange
- may cause headache, vertigo, hepatic toxicity
- monitor renal function

Phenytoin

Generic Name

phenytoin

Trade Name

Dilantin

Indication

tonic clonic seizures, arrhythmias, neuropathic pain

Action

interferes with ion transport, shortens action potentials and decreases automaticity

Therapeutic Class

antiarrhythmics, anticonvulsants

Pharmacologic Class

hydantoins

Nursing Considerations

- use cautiously in all patients
- can cause suicidal thoughts, ataxia, extraparymidal symptoms, hypotension, tacchycardia, gingival hyperplasia, nausea, rash, drug induced hepatitis, aggranulocytosis, Steven's johnson syndrome
- concurrent administration of enteral feedings may decrease absorption
- monitor for hypersensitivity
- assess seizures
- assess hemodynamics
- monitor serum phenytoin levels
- therapeutic levels 10-20 mcg/mL

Procainamide

Generic Name

procainamide

Indication

wide variety ventricular and atrial arrhythmias, PAC, PVC, VTach, post cardioversion

Action

decreases excitibility and slows conduction velocity

Therapeutic Class

antiarrhythmic (Class IA Na Channel Blocker)

Nursing Considerations

- may cause ventricular arrhythmias, seizure, asystole, heart block
- monitor EKG continuously may cause widening of QRS complex
- may cause hypotension keep patient supine
- monitor for signs of agranulocytosis monitor CBC frequently
- can cause drug induced lupus syndrome

Promethazine

Generic Name

promethazine

Trade Name

Promethacon

Indication

allergic reactions, nausea and vomiting, sedation

Action

blocks the effects of histamine, histamine plays a role in the immune response. also plays an inhibitory role on the chemoreceptor trigger zone in the medulla leading to an antiemetic effect. possess anticholinergic properties producing CNS depression

Therapeutic Class

antiemetic, antihistamine, sedative/hypnotic

Pharmacologic Class

phenothiazine

Nursing Considerations

- IV administration may cause damage to tissue, hypertension, impaired liver function
- Monitor for neuroleptic malignant syndrome, confusion, sedation
- May cause CNS depression
- assess sedation level and anticholinergic effects

Propofol

Generic Name

propofol

Trade Name

Diprivan

Indication

anesthesia, induction, sedation,

Action

hypnotic, produces amnesia

Therapeutic Class

general anesthetic

Pharmacologic Class

none

Nursing Considerations

- use cautiously with CVD, lipid disorder, increased ICP
- can cause apnea, bradycardia, hypotension
- burning and pain at insertion site
- can turn urine green
- assess respiratory status and hemodynamics
- maintain patent airway
- assess level of sedation

Propranolol

Generic Name

propranolol

Trade Name

Inderal

Indication

hypertension, angina, arrythmias, cardiomyopathy, alcohol withdrawal, anxiety

Action

blocks Beta 1&2 adrenergic receptors

Therapeutic Class

antianginal, antiarrhythimic (class II beta blockers), antihypertensive, headache suppressant

Pharmacologic Class

beta blocker

Nursing Considerations

- Contraindicated in CHF, pulmonary edema, cardiogenic shock, bradycardia, heart block
- monitor hemodynamic parameters (HR, BP)
- May cause bradycardia, CHF, pulmonary edema
- Masks symptoms associated with diabetes mellitus
- advise to change positions slowly to prevent orthostatic hypotension
- instruct patient on how to take blood pressure
- stopping abruptly may result in life threatening arrhythmias
- monitor daily intake and output
- advise patient to notify physician for difficulty breathing

Propylthiouracil

Generic Name

propylthiouracil

Trade Name

PTU

Indication

hyperthyroidism

Action

inhibits thyroid hormones

Therapeutic Class

Antithyroid Agent

Pharmacologic Class

none

Nursing Considerations

- hepatotoxicity, nausea, vomiting, agranulocytosis
- monitor symptoms of hyperthyroidism
- monitor for hypothyroidism
- monitor WBC and liver function tests
- weight patient frequently
- may cause leukopenia, thrombocytopenia, jaundice
- take with meals

Quetiapine

Generic Name

quetiapine

Trade Name

Seroquel

Indication

schizophrenia, depressive disorder, mania

Action

dopamine and serotonin antagonist

Therapeutic Class

Antipsychotic, mood stabilizers

Pharmacologic Class

none

Nursing Considerations

- may cause neurolyptic malignant seizures, dizziness, palpitations, weight gain, anorexia
- don't use with CNS depressants
- assess weight frequently
- monitor liver function test and CBC
- may increase cholesterol

Ranitidine

Generic Name

ranitidine

Trade Name

Zantac

Indication

duodenal ulcers, GERD, heartburn, esophagitis, GI bleed

Action

inhibits action of histamine in gastric parietal cells, decreases gastric acid secretion

Therapeutic Class

antiulcer agents

Pharmacologic Class

histamine H2 antagonists

Nursing Considerations

- may cause arrhthmias, agranulocytosis, aplastic anemia, confusion
- assess abdominal pain
- monitor for blood in stool
- monitor CBC

Rifamipin

Generic Name

rifampin

Trade Name

Rimactane

Indication

tuberculosis

Action

inhibits RNA synthesis

Therapeutic Class

Antitubercular

Pharmacologic Class

rifamycins

Nursing Considerations

- can turn body fluids red
- may cause diarrhea, nausea, vomiting, confusion
- assess lung sounds and sputum characteristics
- evaluate renal and liver function tests
- instruct patient not to skip or double dose

Salmeterol

Generic Name

salmeterol

Trade Name

Serevent

Indication

reversible airway obstruction, exercise induced asthma

Action

bronchodilation through stimulation of beta 2 adrenergic receptors

Therapeutic Class

bronchodilators

Pharmacologic Class

adrenergics

Nursing Considerations

- instruct patient to avoid excessive use
- can cause headache palpitations tachycardia, abdominal pain, paradoxical bronchospasm
- beta blockers and decrease effectiveness
- assess respiratory status
- may increase glucose levels

Sertraline

Generic Name

sertraline

Trade Name

Zoloft

Indication

major depressive disorder, OCD, anxiety

Action

inhibits uptake of serotonin

Therapeutic Class

Antidepressant

Pharmacologic Class

SSRI

Nursing Considerations

- don't use with MAOIs
- can cause neurolyptic malignant syndrome, suicidal thoughts, drowsiness, insomnia, diarrhea, dry mouth, tremors, serotonin syndrome, sexual dysfunction
- monitor mood changes in patient
- takes 1-4 weeks for therapy to be effective.

Spironolactone

Generic Name

spironolactone

Trade Name

Aldactone

Indication

potassium loss, hypertension, edema, CHF

Action

inhibits sodium reabsorption while sparing potassium and hydrogen

Therapeutic Class

Diuretics

Pharmacologic Class

potassium sparing diuretics

Nursing Considerations

- contraindicated with hyperkalemia
- monitor intake and output
- monitor blood pressure
- monitor potassium levels and renal panel

Streptokinase

Generic Name

streptokinase

Trade Name

Streptase

Indication

pulmonary embolism, DVT, occluded lines, arterial thrombus

Action

converts plasminogen to plasmin which degrades fibrin clots

Therapeutic Class

Thrombolytic

Pharmacologic Class

plasminogen activators

Nursing Considerations

- contraindicated with active bleeding, hypersitivity, bronchospasm, intracranial hemorrhage, hypotension
- begin therapy as soon as possible
- monitor vital signs continuously
- monitor closely for bleeding
- monitor hemodynamics
- avoid invasive procedures

Sucralfate

Generic Name

sucralfate

Trade Name

Carafate

Indication

management of GI ulcers, GI injury prevention from high dose aspirin and NSAID treatment

Action

reacts with gastric acid to form a paste that adheres to ulcer

Therapeutic Class

antiulcer agent

Pharmacologic Class

GI protectant

Nursing Considerations

- use caution in renal failure patients
- concurrent use of antacids may decrease the effect of sucralfate - administer 30 min before or after
- administer on empty stomach 1 hour before meals

Tertbutaline

Generic Name

terbutaline

Trade Name

Brethaire

Indication

asthma, COPD, preterm labor

Action

produces bronchodilation

Therapeutic Class

bronchodilators

Pharmacologic Class

adrenergics

Nursing Considerations

- may cause nervousness, restlessness, tremors
- beta blockers can reduce effect
- assess respiratory status
- monitor maternal/fetal vital signs if using for preterm labor
- monitor for hypoglycemia
- may cause decreased potassium level

Tetracycline

Generic Name

tetracycline

Trade Name

Doxycycline

Indication

treatment of infection, gonorrhea & syphilis with penicillin allergy, chronic bronchitis

Action

bacteriostatic by inhibiting protein synthesis

Therapeutic Class

anti-infectives

Pharmacologic Class

Tetracyclines

Nursing Considerations

- use caution with liver impairment
- may cause pseudomembranous colitis, diarrhea, nausea, vomiting, photosensitivity, rash
- may increase effects of warfarin
- assess for infection
- obtain culture prior to initiating therapy
- monitor renal and liver labs
- instruct patient to complete entire dose.

Trimethoprim/sulfamethoxazole

Generic Name

trimethoprim/sulfamethoxazole

Trade Name

Bactrim/TMP-SMZ

Indication

bronchitis, UTI, diarrhea, pneumonia, multiple types of infection

Action

bacteriacidal by preventing metabolism of folic acid

Therapeutic Class

anti-infectives, antiprotozoals

Pharmacologic Class

folate antagonists, sulfonamides

Nursing Considerations

- may cause renal damage, Steven Johnsons Syndrome - rash, pseudomembranous colitis, nausea, vomiting, diarrhea, rash, agranulocytosis, aplastic anemia, phlebitis
- contraindicated with sulfa allergies
- monitor CBC
- obtain cultures prior to initiating therapy
- monitor intake and output
- instruct patient to complete dose

- drink 8-10 glasses of water

Vancomycinn

Generic Name

vancomycin

Trade Name

Vancocin

Indication

life threatening infections,

Action

bacteriacidal

Therapeutic Class

anti-infectives

Pharmacologic Class

none

Nursing Considerations

- can cause ototoxicity, nausea, vomiting, nephrotoxicity, anaplhylaxis, red-man syndrome
- assess for infection
- obtain culture prior to initiating therapy
- monitor blood pressure

Vasopressin

Generic Name

Vasopressin

Trade Name

Pitressin

Indication

management of diabetes insipidus, VT/VF unresponsive to initial shock, GI hemorrhage

Action

increases water permeability of the kidney's collecting duct and distal convoluted tubule leading to water retention, also increases peripheral vascular resistance leading to increased BP

Therapeutic Class

hormone

Pharmacologic Class

antidiuretic hormone

Nursing Considerations

- use caution with HF and CV disease
- contraindicated in renal failure and hypersensitivity to pork
- monitor BP, HR, and EKG during therapy
- monitor urine specific gravity and osmolality
- weigh patient and assess for edema
- monitor electrolyte panel
- do not use with alcohol

Verapamil

Generic Name

verapamil

Trade Name

Isoptin

Indication

hypertension, angina, SVT, migraine

Action

prevents transport of calcium, leading to decreased contraction, decreases SA and AV node conduction

Therapeutic Class

antianginals, antiarrhythmics, antihypertensives, vasccular headache suppresants

Pharmacologic Class

Ca Channel Blocker

Nursing Considerations

- don't use with 2nd and 3rd degree heartblock
- don't use with systolic BP < 90
- may cause anxiety, confusion, cough, dyspnea, arrythmias, CHF, bradycardia, hypotension, elevated liver enzymes, Steven's johnson syndrome, hyperglycemia, gingival hyperplasia
- grapefruit juice can increase effects
- can increase levels of digoxin
- monitor heart rhythm, intake and output, blood pressure
- assess angina

Warfarin

Generic Name

warfarin

Trade Name

Coumadin

Indication

venous thrombosis, pulmonary embolism, A-fib, myocardial infarction

Action

disrupts liver synthesis of Vitamin K dependent clotting factors

Therapeutic Class

Anticoagulant

Pharmacologic Class

coumarins

Nursing Considerations

- contraindicated with bleeding, severe hypertension
- can cause bleeding
- aspirin and NSAIDs can increase risk of bleeding
- azole antifungals increase effects of warfarin
- cimetadine(Tagamet) increases warfarin levels
- obtain full history of supplements and herbs
- large amounts of vitamin K may antagonize effects of warfarin
- assess for signs of bleeding
- therapeutic levels: PT 1.3-1.5, INR 2.5-3.5
- instruct patient to report any signs of bleeding
- patient should not drink alcohol
- bleeding times need to be monitored frequently

Common Medication Classes

ACE Inhibitors

Angiotensin-converting enzyme (ACE) inhibitors are a type of drug class most often used to relax blood vessels. ACE Inhibitors work by causing the body to block the production of a hormone knows and angiotensin II by inhibiting the angiotensin-converting enzyme. Angiotensin II, found naturally in the body, constricts blood vessels and releases a hormone that elevates blood pressure, making the heart work harder. The hormone also reduces the amount of water re-absorbed by the kidneys. These drugs also work in the body by decreasing the conversion of angiotensin I to angiotensin II, hence their name. Decreasing levels of angiotensin II causes the blood vessels to dilate and for less water to be put back into the blood by the kidneys, reducing blood pressure. Some common ACE Inhibitors include: captopril, enalapril, fosinopril, imidapril, lisinopril, perindopril, ramipril, and trandolapril.

ACE Inhibitors are typically taken once a day and may be prescribed by a doctor for some of the following conditions: high blood pressure (hypertension), heart failure, kidney disease, diabetes, heart attacks, coronary artery disease, scleroderma, and migraines. Doctors may prescribe calcium channel blockers and diuretics in addition to drugs in this class. ACE inhibitors should not be taken by women that are pregnant or planning to become pregnant, as they can cause birth defects. The safety and efficacy of this drug class for children are not known and is not commonly prescribed for children.

ACE Inhibitors are commonly prescribed by doctors because of their uncommon and mild side effects. Side effects may include: dry cough, increased blood potassium levels (hyperkalemia), fatigue, dizziness, headaches, rapid heartbeat, and fainting. In rare cases, particularly with those of African descent and tobacco users, use of ACE Inhibitors has been tied to angioedema, or swelling of the tissue. This can be life threatening if the tissues in the throat swell. Repeated use of NSAIDs (nonsteroidal anti-inflammatory drugs) such as Ibuprofen, Advil, and Motrin IB in addition to naproxen (Aleve) can decrease the effectiveness of ACE Inhibitors.

Questions about ACE Inhibitors:

1. What are some of the contraindications of the use of ACE Inhibitors?
2. How do ACE Inhibitors specifically work to lower blood pressure?
3. What are some potential side-effects that should be monitored in patients taking ACE Inhibitors?

Angiotensin II Receptor Blockers

The cardiovascular system reacts in various ways to the natural Angiotensin II in the body. Angiotensin II is a potent chemical that causes contraction of muscles that surround blood vessels. Blood vessels narrow. The narrowing causes increased blood pressure. The heart is forced to work harder. Amounts of water and sodium caused by a hormone that Angiotensin II starts to release also cause increased blood pressure. Blood vessels and heart walls thicken and stiffen due to Angiotensin II.

How the Drug Works in the Body

Angiotensin II receptor blockers relax blood vessels. The heart pumps blood more effortlessly. As the blood vessels relax, blood pressure lowers. The use of Angiotensin II receptor blockers blocks the action of Angiotensin II. The blockers prevent binding to receptors on blood vessels. Blood vessels widen or dilate.

Listed here are conventional Angiotensin II receptor blockers and their trade names. The condition being treated and the health of the patient determine the best choice.

- Candesartan (Atacand)
- Irbesartan (Avapro)
- Olmesartan (Benicar)
- Losartan (Cozaar)
- Valsartan (Diovan)
- Azilsartan (Edarbi)
- Temisartan (Mecardis)
- Eprosartan (Teveten)

Indications for Use

Conditions that merit prescribing Angiotensin II receptor blockers include thickening and hardening of the skin, known as scleroderma. They are beneficial when prescribed for chronic kidney diseases, diabetic renal failure, heart failure and high blood pressure. Kidney disease progression due to diabetes or high blood pressure diminishes. Reduced risk of stroke or diabetes prevention is possible in high blood pressure patients. Avoiding atrial fibrillation recurrence may be a benefit of Angiotensin II. Patients who cannot tolerate ACE (angiotensin-converting-enzyme) inhibitors are often prescribed Angiotensin II receptor blockers because they produce similar effects.

Side Effects

Very few people suffer from Angiotensin II receptor blocker side effects. Those who do, report bouts of

· Diarrhea
· Leg and back pain
· Nasal congestion
· Lightheadedness
· Dizziness
· Headaches.

Some people taking Olmesartan reported sprue-like enteropathy that is an intestinal problem. Other rare, but serious, side effects are angioedema (localized tissue swelling), white blood cell drop, allergic reaction, liver failure, and kidney failure. Women planning a pregnancy, or are already pregnant should not take Angiotensin II receptor blockers. They are a possible cause of birth defects.

Questions:

When are Angiotensin II receptor blockers prescribed?
How do Angiotensin II receptor blockers work?
What are possible side effects of Angiotensin II receptor blockers?

Antianginals

Antianginals are used to manage the pain of angina. They act by either reducing the oxygen needs of the heart or by improving the oxygen flow to the heart, or both. There are three major classes of antianginals and three different types of angina. Stable angina is caused by a partial occlusion of a coronary artery. Unstable angina is due to the rupture of an atherosclerotic plaque. Variant angina is due to vasospasm of coronary arteries.

Beta-adrenoreceptor antagonists

These drugs reduce the heart rate, which reduces the metabolic needs of the heart. They are used to prevent attacks of stable angina due to exertion. They block the beta receptors and keep the heart rate down below the point at which pain occurs.

Beta blockers are indicated as a first-line treatment for stable angina. They are often used in combination with calcium blockers. Beta blockers are contradicted in variant angina and in people with severe asthma. They should be used cautiously in diabetics because they can cause hypoglycemia.

Organic nitrates

These drugs are vasodilators that improve perfusion of the heart. They stimulate the endothelium-derived relaxing factor that dilates the veins and reduces pressure in the ventricles. Both of these mechanisms of action reduce oxygen requirements of the heart muscle.

Nitrates are taken both for immediate relief of painful stable angina attacks and as maintenance therapy to prevent future attacks. However, long-term maintenance nitrate use may cause increased oxidative stress and endothelial dysfunction and may not be safe.

Calcium antagonists

Calcium blockers, or antagonists, dilate blood vessels, improve heart efficiency and reduce the heart rate. Calcium blockers come in three different classes. Class I blockers have a strong negative inotropic effect. Class II blockers do not affect the conductivity or contractions of the heart. Class III blockers have no inotropic effects.

Calcium blockers are used to treat stable angina and variant angina. For treating stable angina, they can be used alone or in combination with beta blockers.

Long term use of Class I calcium blockers may lead to heart failure.

Study Questions

1. Which class of drug is used to abort angina attacks?
2. Which class of drug can cause hypoglycemia in diabetics?
3. Which two classes of drugs are often used together to treat stable angina?

Antidysrhythmics

Antidysrythmic drugs are commonly used to treat dysrhythmias. A dysrhythmia is an abnormal heart beat, and these drugs can help to correct any abnormalities. There are four different classes of drugs that medical professionals should consider when administering the drugs. Here are some details of the four classes and the contraindications.

Classes of Antidysrhythmic

Class I:

Class I drugs are known for interacting with the sodium channels. This class is further subdivided into a, b, or c class.

Class II:

Class II drugs are beta-blockers and work by reducing the sympathetic nervous system stimulation associated with the heart. Impulses in the heart are also reduced or blocked with impulse and transmissions. They work by blocking the effects of catecholamines. If you need to treat supraventricular tachycardias, these drugs are particularly useful.

Class III:

Class III drugs increase the APD through the prolonging of repolarization. These drugs will block potassium channels, but will not affect the conduction velocity. The combination of these two actions will prevent any re-entrant arrhythmias. "Class III agents have the potential to prolong the QT interval of the EKG."

Class IV:

Class IV drugs inhibit the calcium channels by reducing the movement of calcium ions during action potentials. Cardiac action potential is shortened when the conduction through the AV node is decreased. Adrenergic control of heart rate and contractility is controlled through Class IV drugs, which include verapamil or diltiazem.

Adverse Effects

Some common reactions include nausea, diarrhea, vomiting, blurred vision, and headache. Even some antiarrhythmics are known for causing dysrhythmias. Drug toxicity is another adverse effect. Antidysrhythmic drugs involve circulation, CNS, and the heart.

Contraindications

All known drug allergies should be included in addition to cardiogenic shock, major ECG changes, sick sinus syndrome, and bundle branch block.

Interactions

Anticoagulant activity with warfarin is a strong potential with these types of drugs.

The Benefits of Antidysrhythmics are Far-Reaching

Antidysrythmics are important to any medical professional treating patients with irregular heartbeats and other abnormalities associated with heart rhythms. When used properly the drugs are effective. Consider the use of antidysrhythmics to alleviate symptoms in patients who are experiencing related health conditions.

Antiemetics

Medications that help to control nausea and vomiting from a variety of illnesses and conditions are called antiemetics. These medications help to calm the sensations that lead to repeated vomiting and that can lead to fluid loss and severe dehydration. However, these drugs do not treat the underlying medical condition that is causing the nausea and vomiting. A number of different drug classes are used to control nausea and vomiting, including dopamine antagonists, anticholinergics, antihistamines and others.

How Antiemetic Medications Work

Nausea and vomiting are caused by stimulation of the vomiting center in the medulla of the brain. Each class of antiemetic drug works in a different way:

· Anticholinergics – These drugs reduce the action of acetylcholine at the muscarinic receptor of the brain. Dimenhydrinate, diphenhydramine, scopolamine and meclizine are examples of these medications.

· Antihistamines – These drugs inhibit the action of histamine at the H1 receptor in the brain. Metroclopromide, promethazine and doxylamine are examples of these drugs.

· Dopamine antagonists – These drugs work by minimizing the effect of dopamine at the D2 receptor in the chemoreceptor trigger zone of the medulla. Prochlorperazine, chlorpromazine and phenothiazine are examples of this type of medication.

Indications For Use

Antiemetic medications are used for a number of conditions. They are frequently used for severe nausea and vomiting that occurs with pregnancy. Antiemetics are also useful in controlling symptoms of gastrointestinal problems caused by viruses, food poisoning or other issues. Antiemetics are important medications for relieving the nausea and vomiting related to chemotherapy and other cancer treatments. Nausea and vomiting can also occur after surgery, as a result of the effects of anesthesia.

Side Effects

Most side effects from antiemetic medications are minor and are outweighed by the value of the medication for patients. Generally, these side effects fade after a period of use. Side effects include:

· Dry mouth

· Sensitivity to sunlight

· Stuffy nose

· Constipation

However, if more severe side effects, the patient should receive further medical attention immediately:

· Hives

· Fever

· Swelling of lips

· Vision problems

· Uncontrollable facial or body movements

· Fainting

· Trembling

· Sweating

· Problems with breathing

· Seizures

· Loss of bladder control

Anticoagulants

Anticoagulants are used to prevent clots from forming in the blood. Clots can lead to strokes, pulmonary embolisms, heart attacks and deep vein thrombosis. Anticoagulants can be categorized into four main groups.

Vitamin K Antagonists

These anticoagulants act to block vitamin K from modifying certain proteins essential in clotting. Without the action of vitamin K these proteins cannot bind calcium and therefore cannot function. These drugs take several days before they become effective and are only used as long-term anticoagulant maintenance therapy. The most commonly-used drug in this class is coumarin (warfarin).

Heparin

Heparin acts indirectly to block thrombin by activating antithrombin III and blocking the function of factor Xa. Regular heparin requires daily monitoring of blood chemistry to confirm the correct dose is being used. Low-molecular-weight heparins have a better anticoagulant function and do not require daily blood monitoring.

Thrombin Inhibitors

Drugs in this class prevent thrombin from clotting blood. Thrombin forms clots by cleaving and activating fibrin. It is one of the most important proteins in the clotting cascade.

Factor Xa Inhibitors

Factor Xa is essential in the conversion of prothrombin to thrombin. Drugs in this class block Factor Xa from functioning, and therefore less thrombin is produced. These drugs are primarily used to prevent clots from forming in patients undergoing major elective surgeries, such as joint replacements.

Indications, Side Effects and Interactions

Anticoagulants are indicated for any individual thought to be at higher than average risk of developing a clot. Many medical conditions can increase the risk of clot formation.

A serious, and common, complication of anticoagulant therapy is excessive bleeding. Long-term use of vitamin K antagonists can weaken bones and cause calcification of arteries.

Many medications, herbal preparation and even food can interact with anticoagulants. NSAIDs, grapefruit, St. John's wort and feverfew can all increase the risk of excessive bleeding in patients on anticoagulants. Spinach, avocado and coenzyme Q10 all promote clotting and can interfere with the effectiveness of anticoagulant therapy.

Study Questions

1. What class of drugs includes coumarin?
2. What is the most common complication of anticoagulant therapy?
3. How does heparin act to inhibit blood clotting?

Antidepressants

HOW ANTIDEPRESSANTS WORK IN THE BODY

The medications classified as antidepressants are used to treat a number of symptoms and conditions. These drugs work to create balanced chemical levels in the brain's neurotransmitters, in order to reduce symptoms of depression or anxiety disorders. Neurotransmitters link cells, providing communication within the brain. Neurotransmitters are released by a certain nerve and taken up by others; however, when they are not collected by another nerve, they are taken back by the original nerve - a process called "reuptake". The neurotransmitters commonly linked to depression are serotonin, dopamine and norepinephrine.

TYPES OF ANTIDEPRESSANTS

There are a few main types of antidepressants. These include:

Tricyclic (or tetracyclic) antidepressants (TCAs) - Called cyclic antidepressants in general, and categorized by the number of rings in their chemical makeup; three (tri) or four (tetra). These were among the first antidepressants created, but have been widely replaced by more common types (with less side effects). However, they have been found to be successful in certain cases where other antidepressants were not.

Selective serotonin reuptake inhibitors (SSRIs) - Because these particular antidepressants cause fewer side effects than the others, they are the kind that are most often prescribed.

Monoamine oxidase inhibitors (MAOIs) - The first antidepressants created, but they are being used less often because of the possible side effects and dietary restrictions. Because of the risk of high blood pressure, certain foods that may interact with this medication must be limited.

SIDE EFFECTS

Though they are different types, these antidepressants are used to treat the same disorders and symptoms, and generally have similar side effects. These effects may include: Dry mouth; dizziness; blurred vision; drowsiness; constipation; headache; anxiety; insomnia; nausea or vomiting; sexual dysfunction; seizures; and more. While each type of antidepressant has its own specific side effects, the number is quite small compared to the number that all three types have in common.

INDICATIONS FOR USE

The FDA outlines indications for use (conditions for which they are prescribed to treat) for drugs. Antidepressant indications for use typically include: Anxiety disorders; obsessive-compulsive disorder (OCD); panic disorder (PD); post-traumatic stress disorder (PTSD); anorexia and bulimia; personality disorders; attention deficit hyperactivity disorder (ADHD); and several other disorders and/or conditions.

QUESTIONS

What are the three main types of antidepressants used?
What are the neurotransmitters in the brain that are linked to depression?

Antiplatelet Medications

General Information: Antiplatelet drugs are a class of medications that inhibit thrombus (blood clot) formation.

Indications: Antiplatelet drugs are primarily used to treat and/or prevent thromboembolic ischemic events such as stroke or myocardial infarction. They are commonly prescribed to patients who have had cardiac stents placed. Antiplatelet drugs can be paired with thrombolytic (tPA) and/or anticoagulant medications (heparin, warfarin) either to treat acute events or for long-term prevention.

Commonly used antiplatelet drugs include aspirin (ASA), clopidogrel (Plavix), prasugrel (Effient), dipyridamole (Persantine, Aggrenox), and ticagrelor (Brilinta).

Mechanism of Action: Antiplatelet drugs all work by decreasing the platelets' ability to stick to one another and form a clot, called aggregation. Aspirin indirectly inhibits the production of thromboxane, a substance important for clot formation. Clopidogrel, ticagrelor, and prasugrel all bind to and block a receptor called P2Y12, which is involved in the activation of platelets and cross-linkage with fibrin. It is important to know that some antiplatelet drugs, including aspirin, clopidogrel, and prasugrel, bind irreversibly to the platelet; their effects persist for the 7-10 day lifespan of the cell. Newer drugs like ticagrelor have the advantage of binding reversibly, and their effects will wear off within hours of discontinuation of the medication.

Side Effects and Precautions: Because they decrease the body's ability to form blood clots, antiplatelet drugs make bleeding a serious risk for patients taking them. This is especially true for those who concurrently take NSAIDs, thrombolytics, or anticoagulants. Other side effects vary from drug to drug. Caution should be used in patients with a history of GI bleeds or ulcers, or at other risk for bleeding (recent trauma or surgery). Safety has not been established in pregnant or lactating mothers or children. If patients require surgery, discontinuation of antiplatelet drugs is often recommended 7-10 days prior.

Monitoring: Periodic lab monitoring of bleeding time should be performed during therapy.

Patient Education: Teach patients signs of bleeding including CNS/hemorrhagic stroke symptoms. Ensure that patients understand the need for immediate medical attention if signs or symptoms of bleeding are observed.

Questions:

1. Why would a patient with newly placed coronary stents be prescribed an antiplatelet drug?
2. What are some signs and symptoms of bleeding that patients on antiplatelet drugs should be aware of?
3. Why is it recommended that patients discontinue taking aspirin one week before having surgery?

Benzodiazepines

Benzodiazepines are used as sedatives, hypnotics, anxiolytics, muscle relaxants and anticonvulsants. They act by enhancing the response of gamma-aminobutyric acid-A (GABA-A) receptors to GABA, a neurotransmitter. Neurons affected by benzodiazepines become resistant to excitation. Benzodiazepines come in short-term, moderate-term and long-acting forms. They can be taken orally or in injectable or rectal forms.

Indications

Indications for treatment with benzodiazepines include sedation, seizures, insomnia, anxiety, agitation, alcohol wthdrawal, and muscle spasms. It is unclear if benzodiazepines are safe during pregnancy. Alcohol should be avoided when using benzodiazepines.

In health-care settings, benzodiazepines are commonly used for their sedating properties. They are used in intensive care settings with patients experiencing extreme distress. They are commonly given before medical or dental procedures to relieve anxiety- in this use, they can also cause amnesia, so the patient doesn't recall any unpleasant details of the procedure.

In cases of prolonged seizures, administration of fast-acting benzodiazepines is the treatment of choice.

For occasional insomnia, benzodiazepines are quite effective in inducing sleep and keeping patients asleep. They can also be used for the treatment of acute anxiety or agitation and are commonly used to ease the symptoms of alcohol withdrawal.

Side Effects

The most common side effects of benzodiazepines are drowsiness, dizziness, and decreased alertness. Driving accidents and falls are both possible problems. Less-frequent side effects include nausea, confusion and nightmares.

Safety

Benzodiazepines are considered safe for short-term use, but occasionally some individuals will experience cognitive impairment and disinhibition. Some individuals respond paradoxically to benzodiazepines with agitation and panic. Elderly individuals are more likely to suffer severe side effects, including dementia, in response to benzodiazepines. Long-term use of benzodiazepines is controversial because of the development of physical and mental dependence and withdrawal symptoms if the medication is stopped abruptly. Long-term use can also cause cognitive impairment, depression and anxiety. Many guidelines suggest using benzodiazepines continuously for no longer than two to four weeks. They can be used intermittently for longer periods of time.

Abuse

Benzodiazepines are frequently abused, often in association with other drugs of abuse. An overdose of benzodiazepine can cause deep unconsciousness but is rarely fatal on its own. However, when benzodiazepines are taken along with alcohol or opiates, the risk of a fatal reaction increases exponentially.

Study Questions
1. Which neurotransmitter receptor do benzodiazepines act upon?
2. Why is long-term use of benzodiazepines considered unsafe?
3. What are the most common side effects of benzodiazepines?

Calcium Channel Blockers

Calcium channel blockers, or calcium antagonists, relax and widen blood vessels by acting on the muscle cells in the arterial walls. They do this by preventing calcium from entering the cells of the heart and blood vessels, which in turn lowers blood pressure. Some calcium channel blockers provide the added benefit of also slowing down heart rate, which aside from reducing blood pressure, can also relieve angina (chest pain) and help stabilize an irregular heartbeat.

Calcium channel blockers are available in both short-acting and long-acting forms. The short-acting forms distribute quickly, but their effects only last a few hours. The long-acting forms release the medication more slowly, resulting in a longer lasting effect.

Examples of calcium channel blockers include:

- Isradipine
- Amlodipine (Norvasc)
- Diltiazem (Cardizem, Tiazac)
- Felodipine
- Nicardipine (Cardene SR)
- Verapimil (Calan, Veralan, Covera-HS)
- Nifedipine (Procardia)
- Nisoldipine (Sular)

Calcium channel blockers are prescribed to help treat, prevent, or improve the symptoms of a wide variety of conditions, including:

- Arrhythmia (irregular heartbeat)
- Angina (chest pain)
- Migraine
- Brain aneurysm complications
- A number of circulatory conditions, such as Raynaud's disease
- Hypertension (High blood pressure)
- Pulmonary hypertension (High blood pressure that affects the arteries in the lungs)

Calcium channel blockers might not be as effective in lowering blood pressure as beta blockers, diuretics, or angiotensin-converting enzyme (ACE) inhibitors. Therefore, they are usually not considered a first course of treatment when treating high blood pressure. Calcium channel blockers are oftentimes prescribed along with other blood pressure medications or with statins (cholesterol-lowering drugs).

However, in the case of African-Americans, calcium channel blockers have been shown to be more effective than other blood pressure medications such as ACE inhibitors, angiotensin II receptor blockers, or beta blockers.

Some side effects of calcium channel blockers include:

- Rash
- Flushing
- Fatigue
- Nausea
- Tachycardia (rapid heartbeat)
- Headache
- Dizziness
- Constipation
- Swelling in the lower legs and feet

Certain calcium channel blockers interact negatively with grapefruit juice, the most outstanding interaction occurring while taking Felodipine. Also, some calcium channel blockers can reduce the body's ability to eliminate calcium channel blockers. The medication then builds up in the system which causes serious side effects.

Questions:

What are calcium channel blockers and how do they work?
What are some examples of calcium channel blockers?
How do calcium channel blockers affect the African-American population differently?

Cardiac Glycosides

Cardiac glycosides are a medication made of an organic molecule with a glycoside sugar. The most common one used in medicine is digoxin, also known as digitalis.

Mechanism of Cardiac Glycosides

Under normal conditions in the absence of cardiac glycoside, sodium-potassium pumps import potassium and export sodium. Another pump, the NCX exchanger, imports sodium into the cell and exports calcium. Cardiac glycosides halt the action of the sodium-potassium pump, making sodium build up in the cell. This stops the NCX pump from working because the cell is already hypernatremic. Calcium will then build up and the excess stored in the sarcoplasmic reticulum.

When released on stimulation, this excess calcium will cause a more powerful and rapid contraction. Cardiac glycosides also increase the repolarization phase of myocytes and thus increase the AV node's refractory period. In higher doses, cardiac glycosides may depress the SA node as well, which can be dangerous.

The result is more effective contraction of the heart muscle and a better regulated heart rate. Cardiac glycosides are anti-arrhythmic and increase cardiac output while reducing the heart rate.

Indications for the Use of Cardiac Glycosides

Cardiac glycosides are used mainly for congestive heart failure and atrial fibrillation. They are contraindicated in patients with ventricular fibrillation.

Side Effects

The most serious side effects of cardiac glycosides are arrhythmia, nausea and vomiting, anorexia, and blurry vision. These symptoms may also suggest toxicity. In addition, common side effects include:

- bradycardia
- loss of consciousness
- dizziness
- bleeding problems from liver toxicity
- rash
- petechiae
- abdominal pain

Because cardiac glycosides are used to treat arrhythmias but also can cause or worsen these, it is important for patients to be monitored when treatment is initiated. However, patients should seek medical care immediately if any of these side effects occur, as all can be dangerous to patients with cardiac failure and also may suggest toxicity.

Questions:

What electrolyte imbalance can mimic the effects of cardiac glycosides?

A patient is started on digoxin. A few days later, he calls his nurse to report side effects of edema, anorexia, and constipation. Which of these may suggest cardiac glycoside toxicity?

Diuretics

Diuretics, or water pills, are a classification of drugs used to treat many different conditions. They work by helping to rid the body of sodium and water by making the kidneys excrete more sodium into the urine. The sodium draws water with it from the blood which reduces the amount of fluid flowing through the blood vessels, thus reducing pressure on the artery walls.

The three main types of diuretics are thiazide, potassium-sparing and loop. Each works differently by affecting a different part of the kidneys. Thiazides not only act on the kidneys, but they also help to dilate the blood vessels. Loop diuretics make the kidneys excrete more fluid by interfering with the transport of salt and water across certain kidney cells in a structure known as the Loop of Henle, where the name is taken from. Potassium-sparing diuretics are weak diuretics most often prescribed in combination with thiazide and loop diuretics to help prevent hypokalemia (low blood potassium). Different diuretic types can also be combined into a single tablet.

Common thiazide diuretics include:

- Indapamide
- Chlorothiazide (Diuril)
- Hydrochlorothiazide (Microzide)
- Metolazone (Zaroxolyn)
- Chlorthalidone

Common potassium-sparing diuretics include:

- Spironolactone (Aldactone)
- Triamterene (Dyrenium)
- Amiloride
- Eplerenone (Inspra)

Common loop diuretics include:

- Furosemide (Lasix)
- Bumetanide
- Torsemide (Demadex)
- Ethacrynic Acid (Edecrin)

The type, and combination of diuretics prescribed depends on the patient's overall health and the condition being treated. Aside from high blood pressure,, edema, and glaucoma, diuretics are used to treat, prevent, or improve symptoms in a range of other conditions such as:

- Heart Failure
- Kidney stones
- Polycystic ovarian disease
- Osteoporosis
- Diabetes insipidus
- Hirsutism (Male-pattern hair growth in women)

Diuretics are usually well tolerated but they do have some side effects, the most common being frequent urination with the use of loop diuretics.

Other possible side effects include:

- hypokalemia (low blood potassium) with potassium-sparing use
- hyperkalemia (high blood potassium) with thiazide use
- Hyponatremia (low sodium in the blood)
- Headaches
- Dizziness
- Muscle cramps
- Increased blood sugar or cholesterol
- Increased thirst
- Joint conditions such as gout
- Impotence
- Rashes
- Gynecomastia (enlargement of the breasts in men)

Questions:

What are the three main types of diuretics and how does each one work?
What conditions do diuretics treat?
What possible side effects are associated with the use of diuretics?

Insulin

Insulin is one of most important hormones in the human body. It helps to regulate the metabolism of carbohydrates and fats that are consumed. When insulin is not produced in the body or is not produced in sufficient quantities, diabetes mellitus can result, a serious metabolic disease that can affect the function of many organs.

What Is Insulin?

Insulin is a protein produced by the human body. The word "insulin" comes from the Latin word meaning "island." Insulin is produced in the pancreas in the islets of Langherans, small areas of the pancreas that contain beta cells that produce the compound. Insulin is produced when carbohydrate foods are ingested and convert to glucose. The insulin helps the body to store and absorb the glucose as it is needed. The insulin in different species of animal is similar to human insulin, but varies in strength. Insulin from pigs is considered to be closest in composition to human insulin.

How Does Insulin Work in the Body?

After eating, glucose in the bloodstream triggers the pancreas to release insulin. The insulin travels to the cells of the body, sending a message to open up to allow the glucose in, so that it can be used for energy or stored for later use. When the body cannot produce its own insulin, or cannot produce enough insulin, it must be introduced artificially into the body to produce this effect.

How Is Insulin Used?

Insulin comes as a solution or in suspension with particles that settle on standing. It must be injected into the body subcutaneously, that is, under the skin. Insulin may come in vials used with syringes; pre-filled disposable devices or cartridges used with insulin pens.

Indications For Use

Insulin is used to regulate blood glucose levels in patients who are not able to produce insulin, such as in Type-1 diabetes, or in patients with Type-2 diabetes whose blood glucose levels cannot be managed with other types of medication.

Side Effects of Insulin

The use of insulin sometimes causes side effects. If side effects are severe, they should be brought to the attention of the physician:

· Redness, swelling or itching at the injection site or on the body

· Skin thickening or depressions in the skin

· Weight gain

· Constipation

Severe side effects that need immediate medical attention include:

· Shortness of breath

· Wheezing

· Dizziness

· Fast heartbeat

· Sweating

· Blurred vision

· Difficulty breathing or swallowing

· Swelling of the extremities

· Muscle cramps

· Weakness

NSAIDs

Mechanism of Action

Nonsteroidal anti-inflammatory agents (NSAIDs) all act to block the cyclo-oxygenase (COX) enzymes. There are two COX enzymes. Both COX enzymes are involved in producing prostaglandins and thromboxanes. COX-1 is present in most tissues, but COX-2 is only produced in inflammatory cells and plays an essential role in inflammation.

Most NSAIDs inhibit both COX enzymes. Their desirable properties are caused by inhibition of COX-2 and most of their side effects are caused by inhibition of COX-1. Inhibition of COX-1 reduces the production of prostaglandins that protect the stomach from acid and support platelet function. As a consequence, all NSAIDs have the potential to cause stomach ulcers and reduce clotting time.

Indications

NSAIDs are used to treat mild to moderate pain and inflammation, and to reduce fevers. Headaches, arthritis pain, and pain associated with minor viral infections are the most common indications for NSAIDs. Low doses of aspirin are also used to reduce the risk of strokes and heart attack by inhibiting clotting of the blood.

Side Effects

The most common side effects of NSAIDs are gastrointestinal in nature and include nausea, reduced appetite, vomiting, diarrhea, and constipation. Some people develop headaches or dizziness. Occasionally swelling of the ankles will occur. More severe side effects include stomach ulcers, kidney failure, liver failure and prolonged bleeding. NSAIDs can also increase the risk of stroke and heart attacks, particularly in individuals already at risk for such conditions. Severe side effects are usually associated with chronic use of NSAIDs.

Warnings and Drug Interactions
Some individuals are allergic to NSAIDs. Anyone with an allergy to one NSAID is likely to be allergic to all NSAIDs.

Aspirin should not be given to children or teenagers with chickenpox or influenza due to the risk of developing Reye's syndrome.

NSAIDs may reduce the effectiveness of diuretics. Because NSAIDs inhibit clotting, they should only be used with care in individuals on anticoagulants such as warfarin.

Administration
NSAIDs are almost always given orally. The dose and frequency of dosing vary by each type of NSAID. Taking the medication with food may reduce the risk of nausea.

Study Questions
1. Which COX enzyme is responsible for protecting the stomach lining?
2. Which NSAIDs can cause stomach ulcers and prolonged bleeding?
3. Who should not be given aspirin?

Opiods

An opioid is within a class of drugs that affect the opioid receptors of the brain. In doing such, the drugs eliminate pain. Many opioid pills exist, and they all resemble morphine in some fashion. Examples of some pills that fall within the opioid class of drugs are Tramadol, Percocet, Methadone and Lortab. Opioid drugs can be classified as Schedule II or Schedule III controlled substances. The drugs are in a pregnancy risk class C, which means they cannot be ruled out as harmful substances to pregnant women.

What Are Opioids Used For?

Various specialists use opioid pills for severe pain that drugs such as acetaminophen and ibuprofen cannot alleviate alone. Most of the aforementioned opiate pills come mixed with acetaminophen or ibuprofen. The mixture of the analgesic and the narcotic gives the patient maximum pain protection. Doctors prescribe opioid pain pills for post-surgery pain, migraine headaches, toothaches, back pain, endometriosis and many other conditions. The government regulates the issuance of such drugs because of the risk for addiction.

How Should Opioids Be Administered?

Specialists usually prescribe opioids to be taken by mouth on an "as needed" basis. The person will normally have to take one to two pills every four to six hours. The individual should not take the opioid pill after the pain subsides. Additionally, a person should not take more than six opioid pills in one day due to the amount of acetaminophen or ibuprofen in the drug. The two substances can cause adverse gastrointestinal effects.

What Are the Side Effects of Opioids?

The most common side effects of an opioid pill are drowsiness and lethargy. Labels often warn patients not to operate vehicles while they are under the influence of such drugs. The reason behind the warning is that people can fall asleep while they are under the influence of opioids.

Nausea is another common side effect that occurs in people who take opioid pills. Some additional side effects include vomiting, itching, sweating, hot flashes and headaches. Such effects do not occur in all patients.

Euphoria is a common side effect of opioid pills. While the effect itself is not dangerous, the potential for addiction comes from it. A person who takes opioid painkillers is under the pretense that he or she is happy, and no pain exists. Therefore, doctors try their best to limit the issuance of such drugs to severe cases.

Statins

Statins reduce cholesterol levels in the body through a process of significant changes.

This drug group targets the liver's cholesterol production, by inhibiting the enzyme HMG-CoA reductase.

This process replaces the HMG-CoA reductase in the liver.

The decreased production of cholesterol initiates two significant occurrences. Supplementary enzymes form and create a protein that significantly increases the production of LDL.

These additional receptors bind with the existing LDL and VLDL in the liver.

The liver digests this fatty substance; reducing cholesterol levels.

Doctors prescribe a statin regimen for people with these conditions.

Atheroma and related diseases, such as heart disease and atherosclerosis

Diabetes

A family history of heart attacks, especially at a young age

Increased age

High cholesterol

There are nine statin drug types.

Atorvastatin [most potent]

Rosuvastatin [most potent]

Cerivastatin

Pravastatin

Lovastatin

Mevastatin

Pitavastatin

Simvastatin

Fluvastatin {least potent}

A single statin drug regimen can successfully reduce cholesterol levels. Sometimes a combination of a statin and niacin [niaspan or niacor] is required, as with these conditions.

High LDL and High Triglycerides
A statin drug and Fibric Acid such as, Fenofibrate {TriCor, Fenoglide} may be useful. There is an increased risk of developing muscle problems.

High Triglycerides only
*Niacin
*Fibric Acid
*Fish Oil, Omega3 fatty acids {Lovaza 2-4 gram doses}

Low HDL
*Niacin {especially if LDL remains high}
*Exercise and weight loss

Statin drug users may experience significant side effects.

Muscle Aches

Pain

Weakness

Neuropathy

Hepatic and Pancreatic dysfunction

Asymptomatic Liver damage

The FDA reports these side effects.

Cognitive impairment [some users report memory loss, forgetfulness, and confusion]

Elevated blood sugar levels.

Lovastatin may interact with other patient medications.

These may indicate the development of severe complications. The physician might request the patient stop taking the medication. If the patient's condition remains unchanged, the doctor can do a more comprehensive evaluation. The physician may order blood tests, a percutaneous muscle biopsy, or genetic tests.

Questions

Can you describe the sequential process of how statins reduce cholesterol levels?
Can you list the types of statin drugs and indicate which ones are the most potent and which are the least potent?

Vasopressors

Vasopressors are compounds used by physicians to force blood vessels to constrict. Many pharmaceuticals have the vasoconstrictive effect, and there are other vasopressors found in nature. Users of vasopressors should be aware that they may cause the blood pressure to rise higher than normal, which could put a person at risk of medical complications. Here are some of the benefits and uses of vasopressors.

Examples of Vasopressors

Caffeine is one of the most common vasoconstrictors. When it's in the body it makes it's own form of epinephrine. They will act on the autonomic nervous system and send the body in a "fight or flight" response due to the stress put on the body.

Common Uses of Vasocompressors

Vasopressors are helpful to manage patients in shock and can help to manage vitals in the operating room. Most vasopressors will be administered by an anesthesiologist, and the patient will be monitored until he or she is stable. Since the drugs are highly specialized, special training is required before administering these drugs.

Characteristics of Vasopressors

Inotropes are commonly used with vasopressors. These compounds are known for influencing muscle contraction. It may cause some muscles to contract and other muscles to relax. Cardiologists use them to stimulate the contraction of the heart's muscle and to increase the force of cardiac contractions. You want to manage the blood pressure while in the operating room to avoid a fatality due to the stresses of surgery.

What Professionals Should Know

All dosages should be carefully measured and administered. Professionals should be concerned with the recommended dosages and the desired effect on the body. All anesthesiologists should be skilled at math and should be able to think quickly and respond during emergencies.

While vasopressors are useful in surgery, they should be used with care. Know all the potential risks involved before administering them. There are some side effects with using natural vasoconstrictors like caffeine, but as long as they are used in moderation, they should not pose health problems. Some people with conditions, such as irritable bowel syndrome, may have other complications with caffeine, but in general it can be useful. Get trained properly and administer vasopressors with caution.

Respiratory Drugs

Drugs that affect the respiratory system can be divided into four general categories.

Antihistamines

Antihistamines, also called H1 blockers, block histamine from binding to receptors. Histamines are released in response to allergens, irritants and general inflammation. When they bind to their receptors, they cause the airways to constrict and release secretions.

Indications for antihistamines include simple allergic reactions, such as allergic sinusitis and urticaria. They can also be helpful for treating rhinitis. Antihistamines are contradicted in pregnancy. They should only be used with caution in individuals with liver or kidney impairment, or with prolonged QT intervals.

Antihistamines come in two classes, first generation and second generation. First-generation drugs have many more side effects due to their stronger anticholinergic effects. The chief side effect to be aware of is sedation.

Decongestants

Decongestants stimulate the alpha-adrenergic receptors, which causes the blood vessels in the mucus membranes to constrict. This reduces the swelling of tissues and the production of secretions. Decongestants come in nasal spray and oral forms.

Decongestants are indicated for rhinitis, sinusitis, allergic reactions, and upper respiratory tract infections. They should only be used cautiously in patients with high blood pressure.

Side effects of decongestants include elevated blood pressure, nervousness and insomnia. Nasal sprays have fewer side effects than oral formulations, but if nasal sprays are used for more than a few days they can cause increased congestion.

Expectorants and Mucolytics

Expectorants act to help individuals clear their respiratory pathways of secretions by increasing the amount of fluid included in the secretions, causing the mucus to become less viscous. The mucolytics also help loosen and break down mucus so it is easier to cough up. They act by directly cleaving chemical bonds in the mucus to make it less viscous.

Indications for mucolytics and expectorants include upper respiratory infections, rhinitis, cystic fibrosis, chronic productive cough and pneumonia.

Side effects of mucolytics are nausea and irritation of the respiratory tract. Side effects of expectorants are nausea and vomiting.

Antitussives

Antitussives act to block the cough reflex. Most antitussives are narcotics that act directly on the nervous system to block coughing without affecting respiration.

Antitussives are indicated in cases of troublesome chronic dry cough. However, caution should be used when administering these drugs because many individuals need to cough to keep their respiratory pathways clear of secretions.

Side effects include drowsiness, nausea, and drying of the mucus membranes.

Questions

What is the primary side effect of first-generation antihistamines?
Can decongestants be given to patients with high blood pressure?
What is the difference between expectorants and mucolytics?

Beta Blockers

Beta blockers, known medically as Beta-adrenergic blocking agents, are typically prescribed for people who have suffered a heart attack or who have high blood pressure. Some common names for these medications include atenolol, acebutolol, bisoprolol, metaprolol, nadalol, and propranolol. This type of medication is usually prescribed after diuretics and other blood pressure medications do not work. They can also be combined with other types of medications called angiotensin-converting enzyme (ACE) inhibitors. According to the American Heart Association, beta blockers can help people live longer after a suffering a heart attack.

What do beta blockers do?

According to the Mayo Clinic, beta blockers block adrenaline or epinephrine. This keeps the heart beating at a slower rate than what a person is used to, and it also keeps the heart from beating as hard as it had been. Beta blockers also open up blood vessels. The combination of opening the vessels and slowing down heart rate keeps blood pressure down.

Beta blockers help reduce systolic blood pressure numbers. These types of medications are prescribed for people who have had a heart attack. They are useful for stopping or lessening angina or chest pain. Beta blockers are also used to control migraines, glaucoma, hyperthyroidism, generalized anxiety disorder, heart failure, and some types of tremors.

What are the side effects of taking beta blockers?

Some of the side effects that people can experience while on this type of medication are fatigue, upset stomach, diarrhea, constipation, and dizziness. Rarer side effects include trouble breathing, depression, loss of sex drive, and trouble sleeping. People who have asthma are not usually prescribed this type of medication due to constriction of the bronchial tubes.

How do beta blockers affect exercise?

Because beta blockers reduce the heart's required oxygen input, people taking beta blockers are able to exercise more regularly without chest pain or irregular heart rhythms. Diabetics should always monitor blood sugar carefully when prescribed beta blockers because the medication can mask the symptoms of low blood pressure like a fast heartbeat.

Speaking to the prescribing physician about exercise and how beta blockers affect the body is always recommended. People who take beta blockers should not stop taking the medication without the advice of a doctor because sudden stopping can cause a heart attack or other heart problems to occur. Taking a beta blocker may help some people tolerate exercise better than they did before they began taking the medicine.

Nursing Assessment

Head-to-Toe Physical Assessment in Pictures

Introduction

This book provides the outline for a basic physical assessment. The head to toe assessment is a fundamental skill in nursing practice and allows the nurse to quickly identify abnormalities in the patient.

This is not intended to be a complete guide to pathophysiology but to provide a framework for completing a thorough head to toe assessment.

Learning to efficiently and quickly complete the exam allows the nurse to understand the patient, their needs, and concerns, and allows the nurse the ability to provide the best possible care.

This book is structured in the recommended order for completing the head to toe assessment. Each section contains a short anatomy section followed by an overview of the assessment technique for the given section. This is followed by a small sample of the abnormal findings the nurse may identify for that body system.

The final chapter of the book includes videos, charts, graphs, and website resources to help you in your assessments.

Head to Toe Assessment Checklist

- General Assessment
- Body Structure/Mobility
- Behavior
- Health History
- Vital Signs
  - Height Weight
  - Pulse Rate
  - Respirations
  - Temperature
  - Blood Pressure
  - Pain
- Integumentary
  - Inspect: color, moisture, hair, rashes, lesions, pallor, edema
  - Palpate: temperature, turgor, lesions, edema, texture
- Scalp
  - Inspect: shape, symmetry
  - Palpate: tenderness, deformity
- Nails
  - Inspect: shape, color
  - Palpate: capillary refill
- Head
  - Inspect: symmetry, shape, size, uniformity
- Neck
  - Inspect: symmetry, lesions, scars
  - Palpate: tenderness, lymph nodes, thyroid gland, TMJ
- Eyes
  - Inspect: interior and exterior, visual fields, acuity, reflexes
- Ears

    - Inspect: color, shape, symmetry, interior inspection
    - Palpate: tenderness, deformity
- Nose
    - Inspect: shape, symmetry, interior inspection
    - Palpate: frontal sinus, maxillary sinuses
- Mouth and Throat
    - Inspect: exterior and interior
- Thorax and Lungs (anterior and posterior)
    - Inspection: respiration quality, symmetry, deformity, tracheal location
    - Palpation: tenderness, fremitus, chest expansion
    - Percussion: percussive tones, diaphragmatic excursion
    - Auscultation: breath sounds and quality
- Heart and Great Vessels
    - Inspection: jugular venous pulse
    - Palpate: pulses, PMI
    - Auscultate: heart sounds (bell and diaphragm)
- Peripheral Vascular System
    - Inspect: color, edema
    - Palpate: temperature, edema
- Abdomen
    - Inspect: discomfort, uniformity, color, symmetry, scars, hernia, peristalsis, pulsations
    - Auscultate: bowel sounds, bruits
    - Percussion: four quadrants, liver, spleen, renal tenderness
    - Palpation: light to deep, liver, spleen, aorta, rebound tenderness, fluid wave
- Musculoskeletal
    - Inspection: asymmetry, deformity, atrophy

    - Palpation: major joints, tenderness, deformity, range of motion
- Neurological
    - Inspect: mental status (health history), cranial nerves, coordination, movement, senses
    - Palpate: motor strength, muscle tone, reflexes, senses
- Genitourinary
    - Inspect: general appearance, lesions, scars
    - Palpate: breast exam, testicular exam, prostate exam, vaginal exam, Pap smear
- Lymphatic
    - Palpate: assess lymph node locations

Integumentary

Anatomy

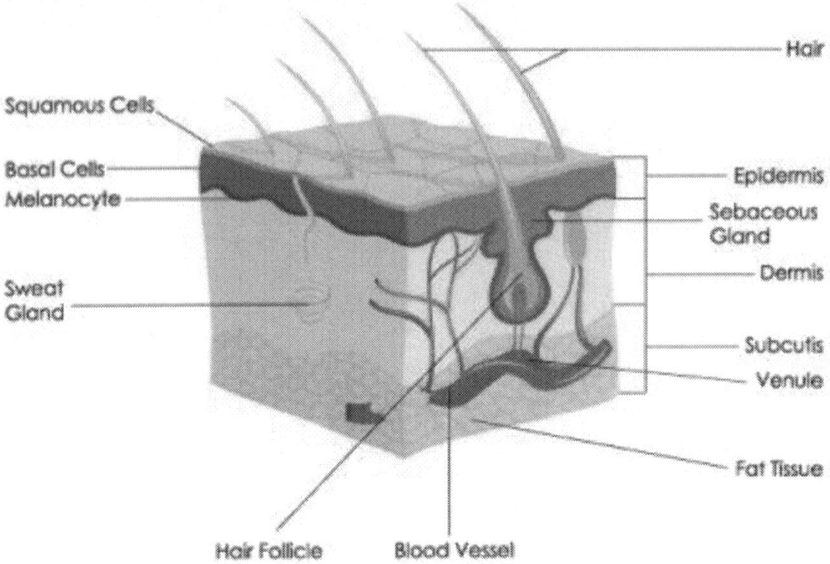

The outermost layer of the skin is called the epidermis. The next layer is the dermis and below that is the subcutaneous layer of fat. Several important glands secrete fluids towards the skin. There are two types of sweat glands. The apocrine sweat glands open into the hair follicles. They respond specifically to emotion or arousal. They begin functioning during puberty. The eccrine sweat glands secrete directly to the skin surface. Their main purpose is the regulation of body temperature. The sebaceous glands secrete a lipid substance into hair follicles.

Hair is a string of proteins that grows from a follicle in the dermis layer of the skin. Hair is made of 3 layers the medulla in the center, the cortex, and then the cuticle.

The nails are made of keratin. The pink color below the nail is due to blood supply to the skin below.

Inspection

Begin your assessment of the skin by looking at the general color or pigmentation of the patient.

The patient's color should be consistent with the genetic makeup of the patient, ranging from pink to dark brown. Darker-skinned people may have areas of lighter pigmentation.

Assess for freckles and birthmarks and use the ABCDE framework to determine abnormality of these markers.

Assess the patient's skin color for any changes in color, also known as pallor, cyanosis, jaundice. It may be more complicated to notice these changes in darker-skinned individuals. The best place to look for these would be nail beds and lips.

Assess hair growth and pattern. Assess for edema.

Palpation

Palpate the skin and assess the temperature. Hypothermia versus hyperthermia. As you feel the skin you should also assess for moisture or diaphoresis.

Assess the mucous membranes for dehydration. The general texture of the skin should be smooth and firm, thickness of the skin should be uniform throughout the body. The heels and palms may be a little bit thicker.

Assess the skin as well for edema, which is fluid accumulation. You can assess for this by palpating on the skin and seeing if there's an imprint left after you lift your hand up. This is known as pitting edema. It could be graded from a scale of +1 to + 4, with +4 being more severe. Edema can mask other more serious signs and symptoms.

Assess the mobility and turgor of the skin. This can be done by pinching the skin up in a fold, upon releasing the fold it should return back to its normal state.

Assess the skin for vascularity and for bruising or lesions. Document their size, color, elevation, general makeup, as well as the location, and make note of any exudate or odor coming from the lesion.

Abnormal Findings

Cyanosis

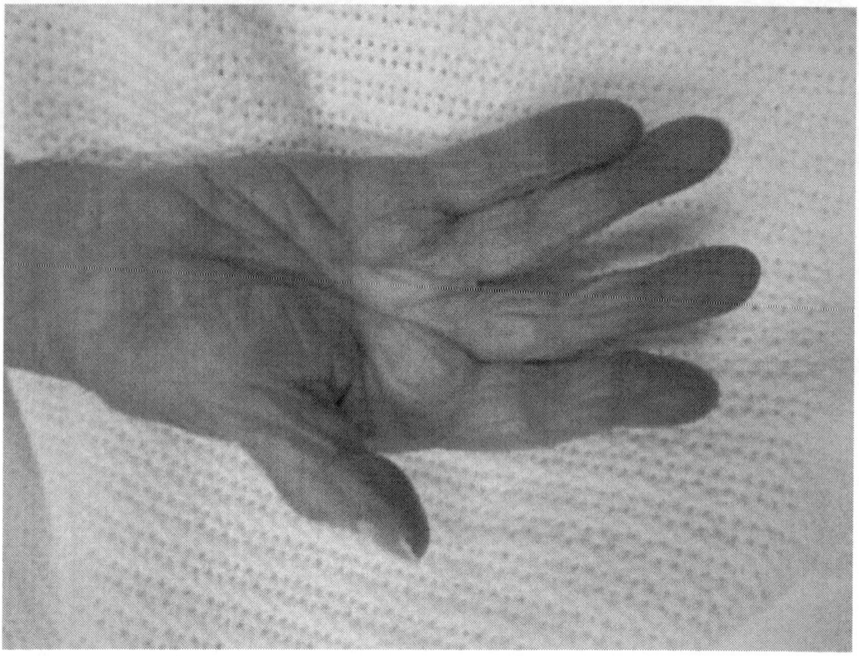

By James Heilman, MD (Own work) [CC BY-SA 3.0 (http://creativecommons.org/licenses/by-sa/3.0)], via Wikimedia Commons

Rash

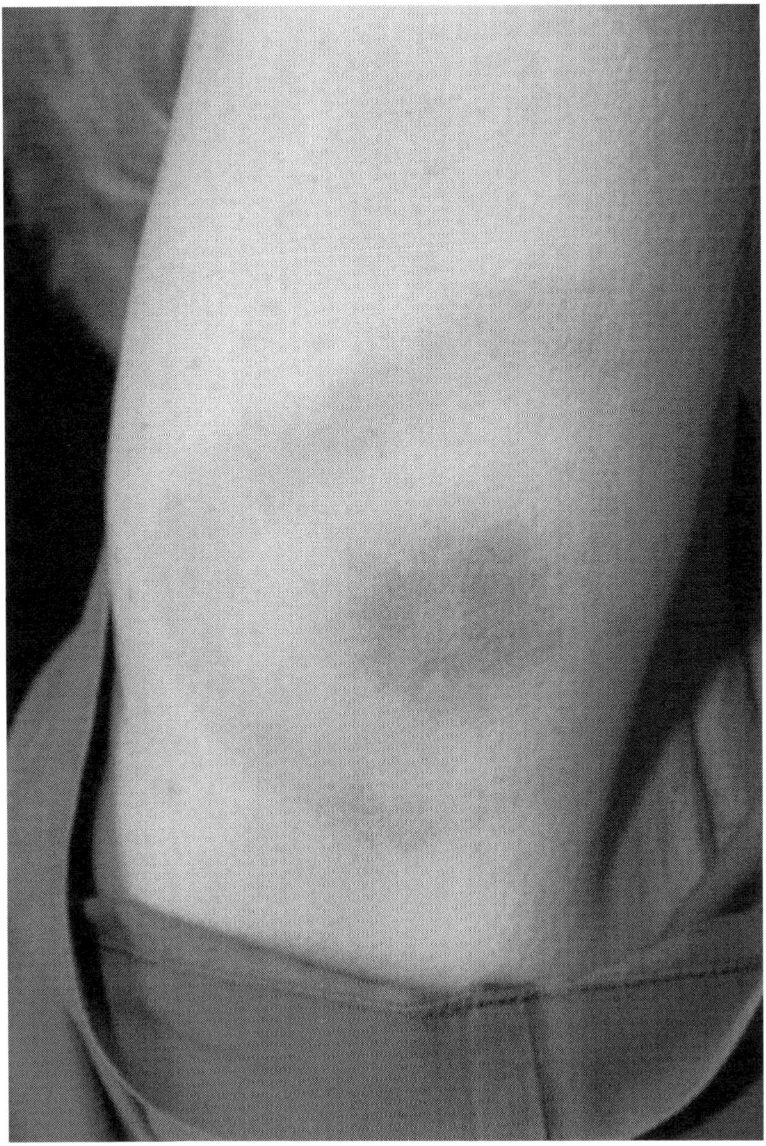

Jaundice

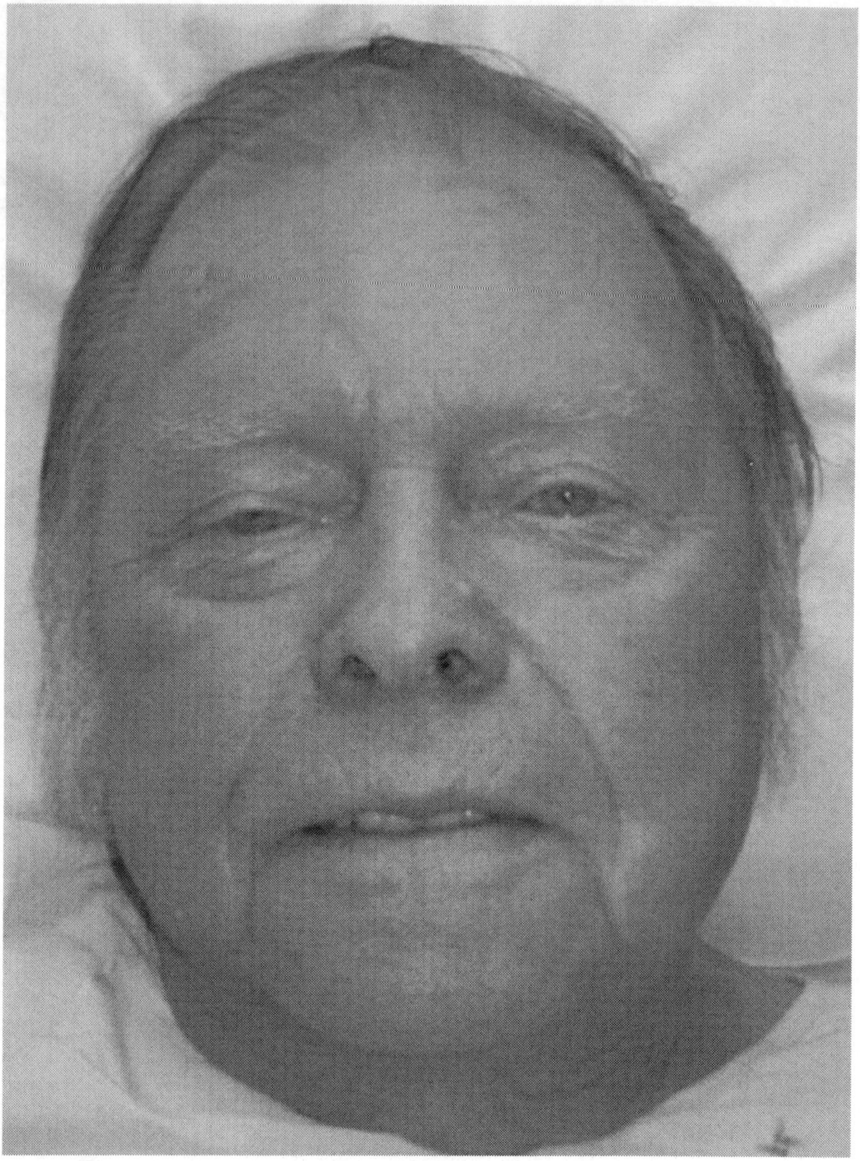

By James Heilman, MD (Own work) [CC BY 3.0 (http://creativecommons.org/licenses/by/3.0)], via Wikimedia Commons

Macule, Patch, Papule, Plaque, Vesicles, Bulla, Fissure, Erosion, Ulcer

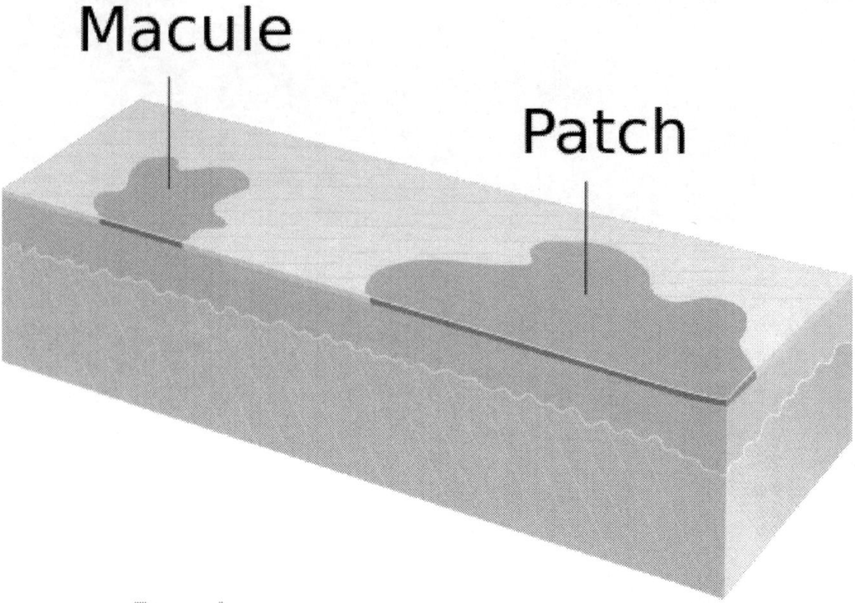

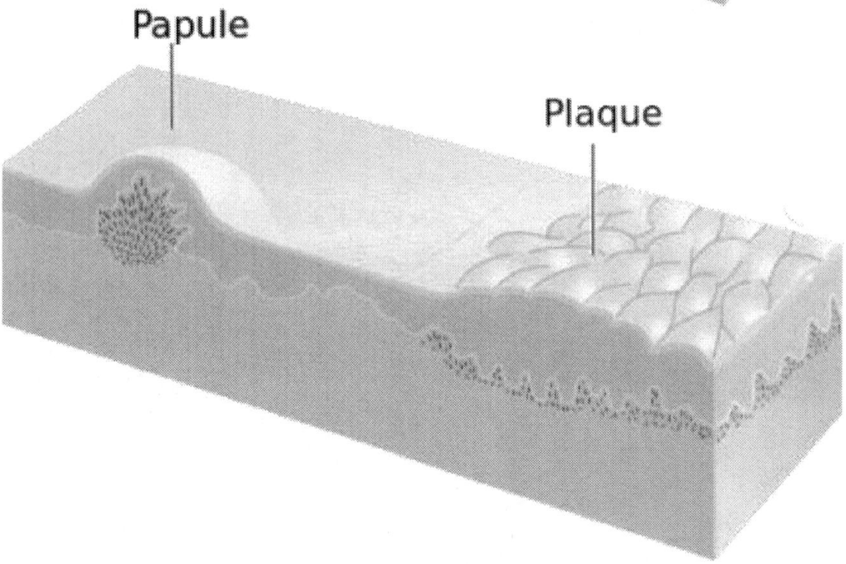

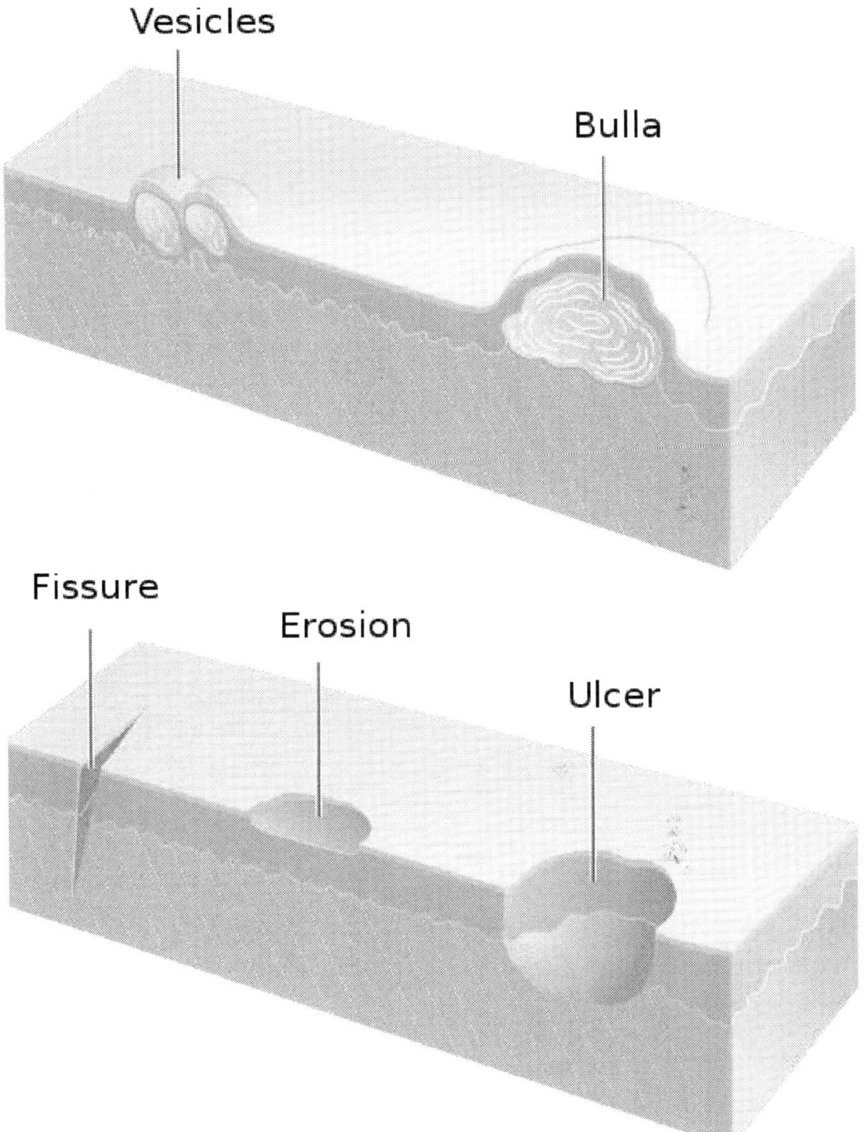
Vesicles
Bulla
Fissure
Erosion
Ulcer

Scalp

Inspection and Palpation

Inspect and palpate the scalp and hair. Assess for the color of the hair and scalp. Assess for shape and symmetry.

Assess the texture of the hair. This can help with understanding nutritional status. Assess for lesions on the scalp and ensure that the patient's scalp is clean.

Nails

Inspection and Palpation

Inspect and palpate the nails. Assess the shape of the nail as well as the color of the nail beds. They should be smooth, clean and round. Assess the surface of the nail to ensure that it is consistent throughout and that the thickness of the nails are uniform.

Lastly, assess for capillary refill. Press on the nail for a second or two, upon removing pressure, color should return to the nail bed within 1 to 2 seconds. Which indicates normal capillary refill.

Abnormal Findings

Clubbing

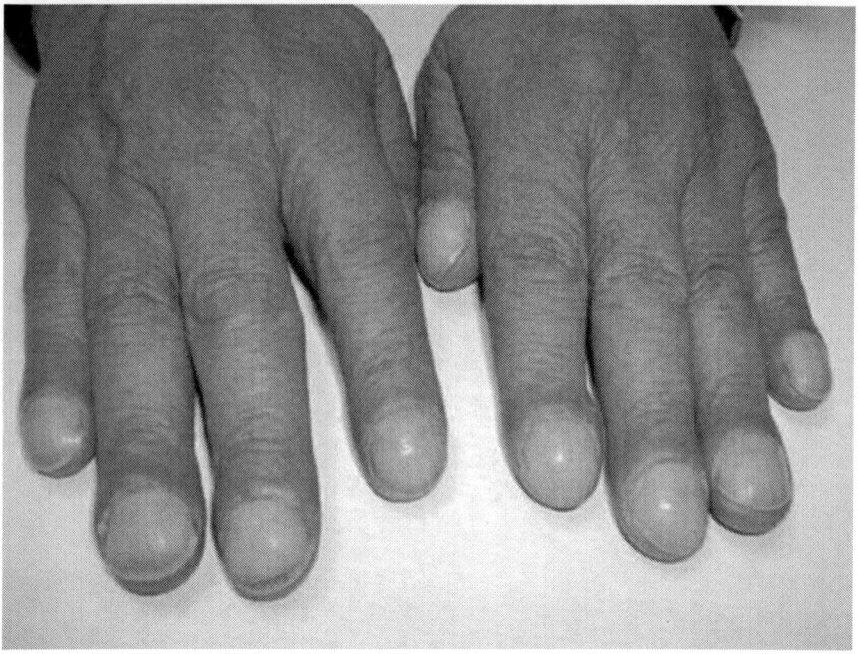

Head

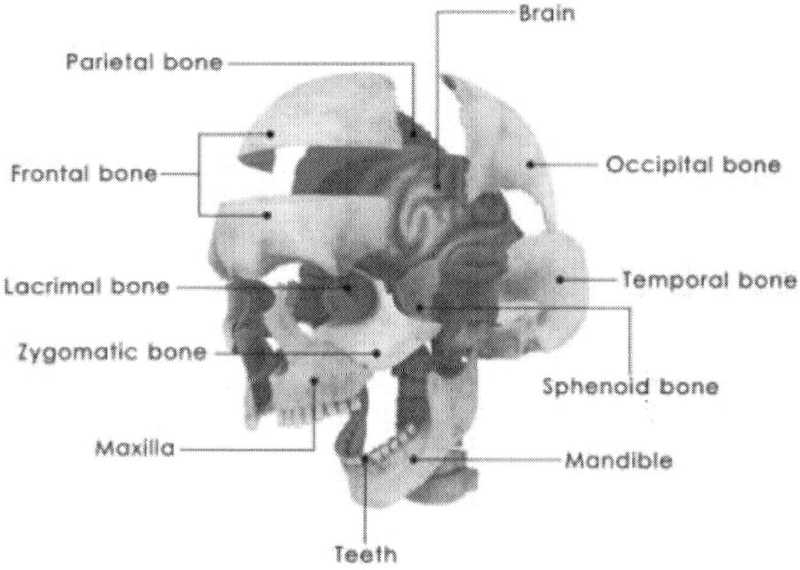

Inspection and Palpation

When assessing the head, start with inspecting and palpating. Inspect the head for general symmetry and appropriate size for the body. The skull should feel symmetrical and smooth. There should be no tenderness on palpation.

Inspect the face for symmetry with the eyebrows, the nose, and the mouth. Make note of any abnormal facial features or swelling or involuntary ticks of the muscles.

Neck

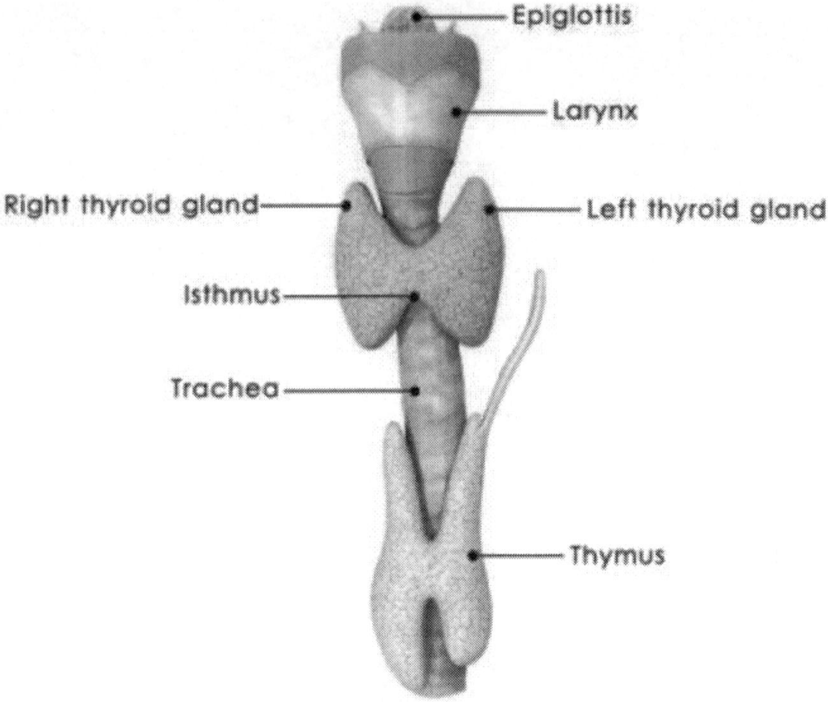

Inspection and Palpation

Inspect the neck for symmetry and ensure that the neck is midline. Assess for neck range of motion, is the patient is able to point the chin down, lift the chin up, and turn from left to right, as well as the shoulders to the ear and extend the head backward. The motions should be smooth and well-controlled.

Assess for lesions or scars.

Palpate the temporal mandibular joint. Palpate for tenderness.

Palpate the lymph nodes. Use a gentle, circular motion to palpate the lymph nodes in front of the ear and within the neck.

Palpate the thyroid gland.

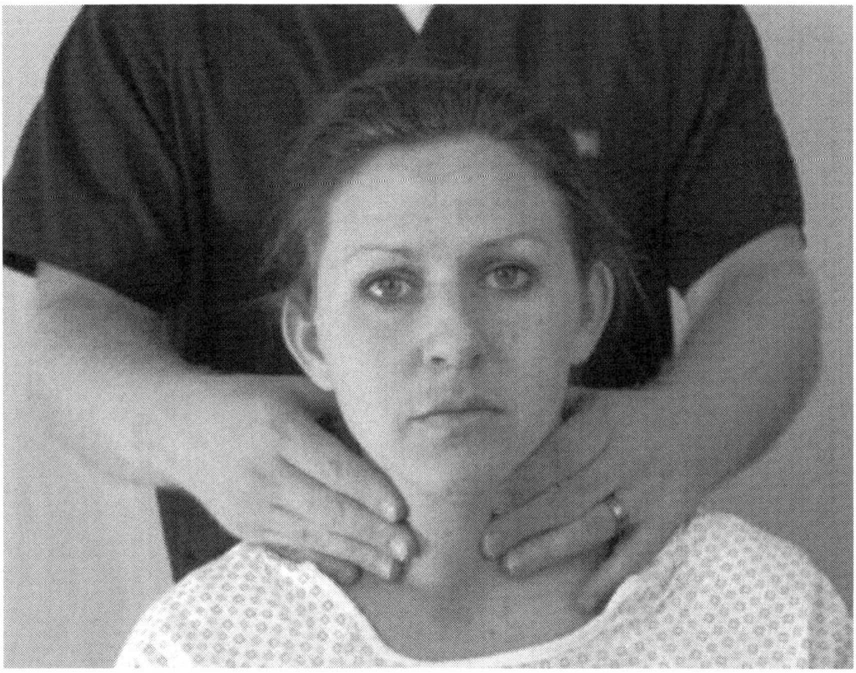

Abnormal Findings

Goiter

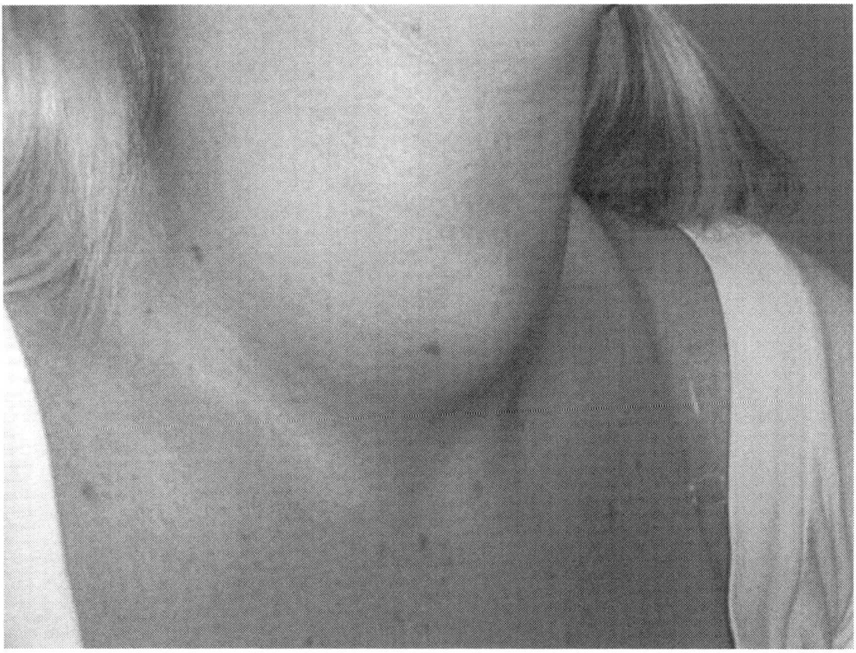

By Drahreg01 (Own work) [GFDL (http://www.gnu.org/copyleft/fdl.html) or CC BY-SA 3.0 (http://creativecommons.org/licenses/by-sa/3.0)], via Wikimedia Commons

Eyes

Anatomy

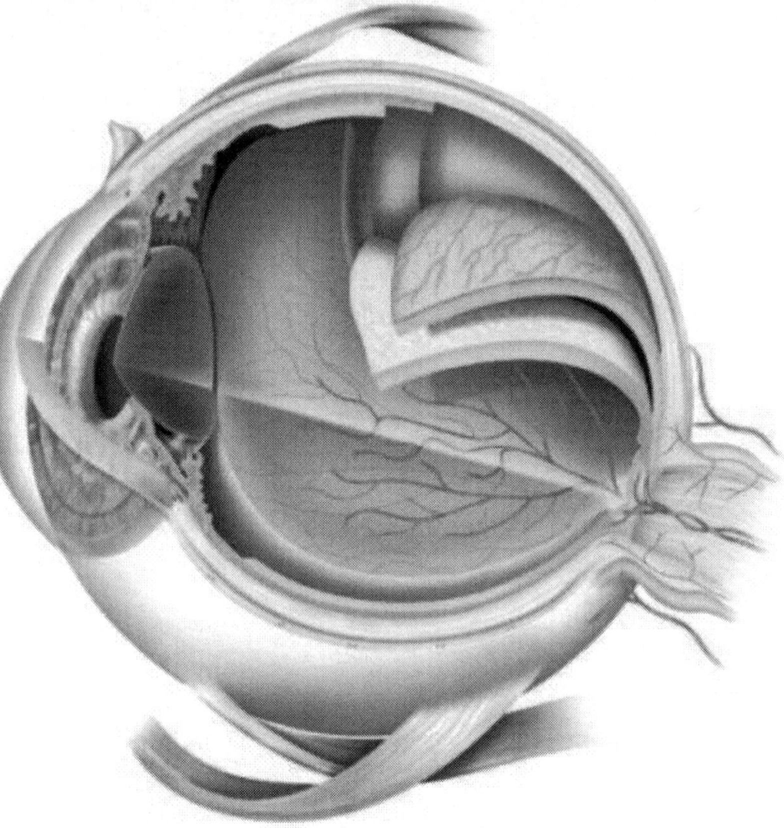

The eye is a sensory organ involved with sight. The eye is protected from external offenses like light or dust by the upper and lower eyelid. The small open space between eyelids is known as the palpebral fissure.

The outermost portion of the eye is the conjuctiva. It lines the inside of the eyelids and the sclera and merges with the cornea which is the outermost covering of the iris and pupil. Behind the cornea is the lens.

A part of the interior of the eye can be visualized with a ophthalmoscope. This area is called the ocular fundus. In this area the optic disc and macula can be seen.

The eye has three lays: sclera just under the conjunctiva, the choroid in the middle, and the retina on the inside. The retina is where light waves are converted into nerve impulses.

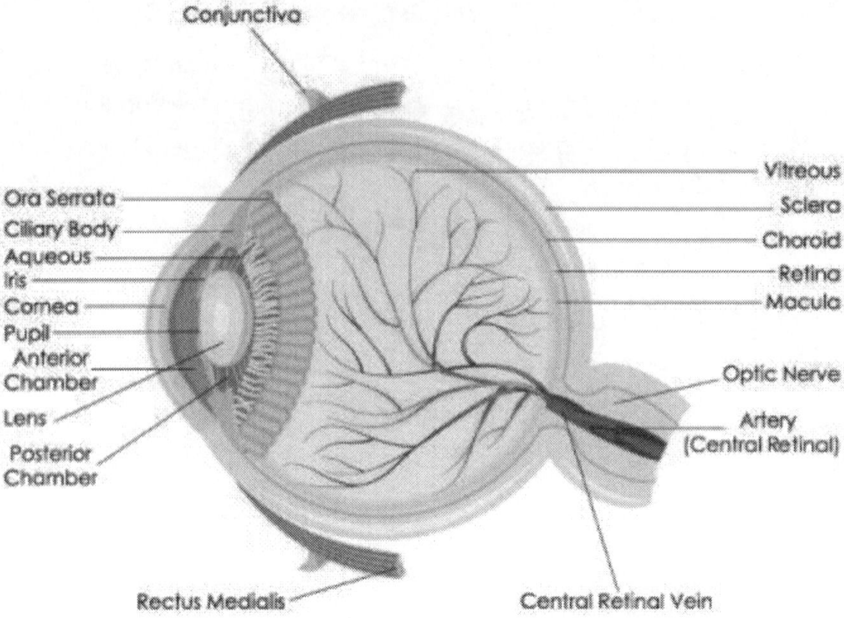

Inspection

When assessing the eyes, inspect the pupils to insure they are equal, round, and reactive to light.

Test for visual acuity with the Snellen chart by having the patient stand 20 feet from the chart. Remove glasses or contact lenses and cover the untested eye.

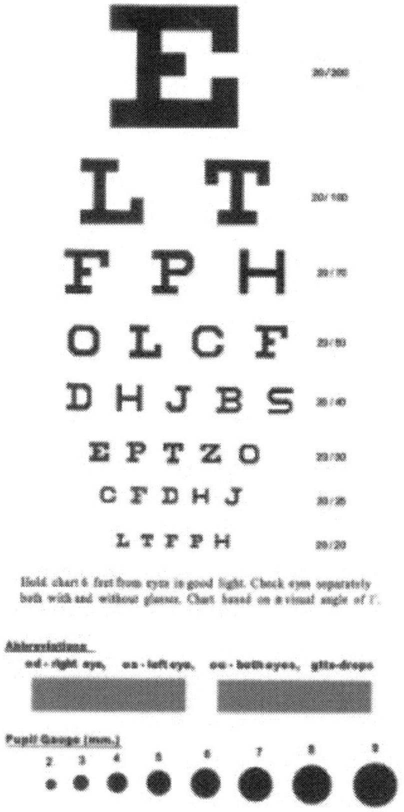

You should test the visual field. Have the patient look in all directions as you move a pencil in those directions. Eye movement should be fluid and well-controlled.

Inspect extraocular muscle function with the 6 cardinal positions. Move your finger in the 6 positions and have the patient follow with their eyes.

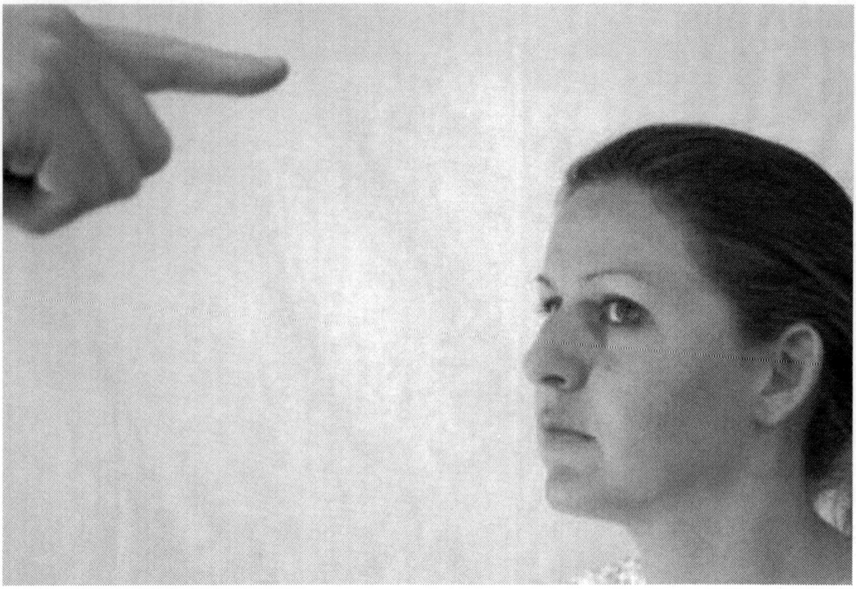

Use the confrontation test to assess visual field. Stand 2 feet away from the patient with a pencil in each hand on either side of the patient. While moving the pencils toward midline have the patient state when they are able to see them.

Assess eyebrows for symmetrical movement bilaterally.

Assess eyelids and lashes, notice any redness, swelling or discharge or lesions.

Assess the general shape of the eye. Inspect the eyeballs for any protrusion or sunken appearance.

Inspect the conjunctiva and the sclera. Ask the patient to look up and while using your thumbs to inspect the conjunctiva and sclera of the patient.

Inspect the interior eyeball structures. Shine a light from side to side and check for smoothness and clarity of the eye.

Inspect the iris and the pupils that the pupils are able to accommodate to light. You should determine that both pupils are equal bilaterally. If the patient has 2 different-sized pupils, this is known as anisocoria.

Inspect the ocular fundus by darkening the room and having the patient remove their glasses. Have the patient look at a specific mark with the eyes fixed while the examiner looks into the eyes to inspect the structures of the ocular fundus, specifically the optic disc retinal vessels, and general background of the macula.

Inspect the color, shape, and margins of the optic disk.

Assess the retinal vessels, the number, the color, and the caliber.

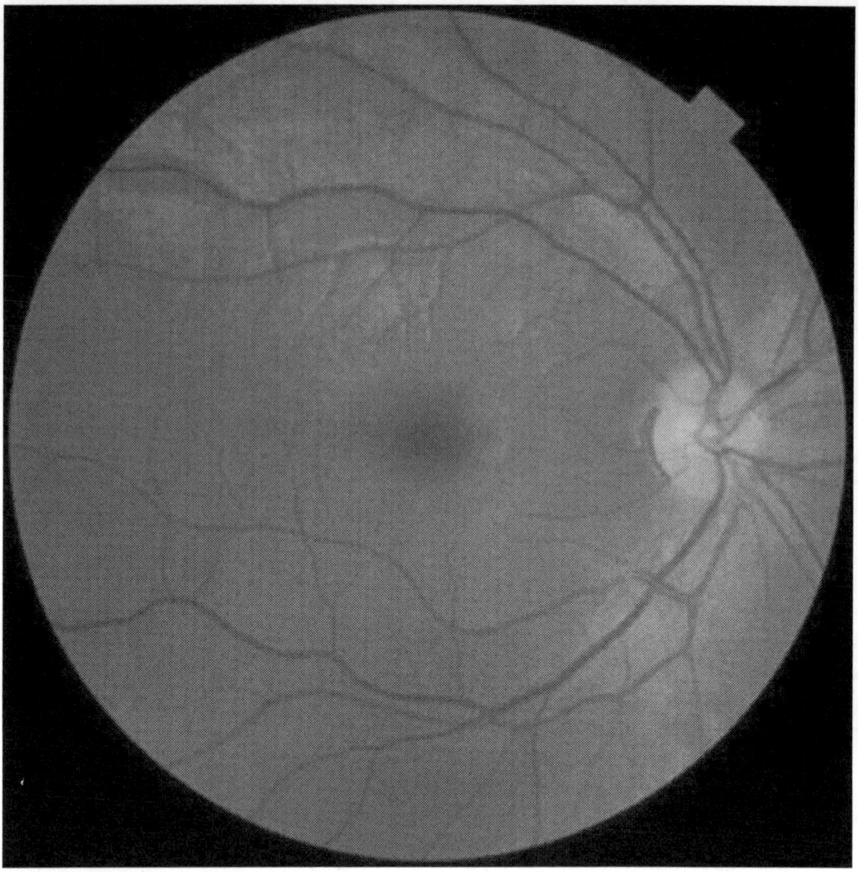

Abnormal Findings

Pinguecula

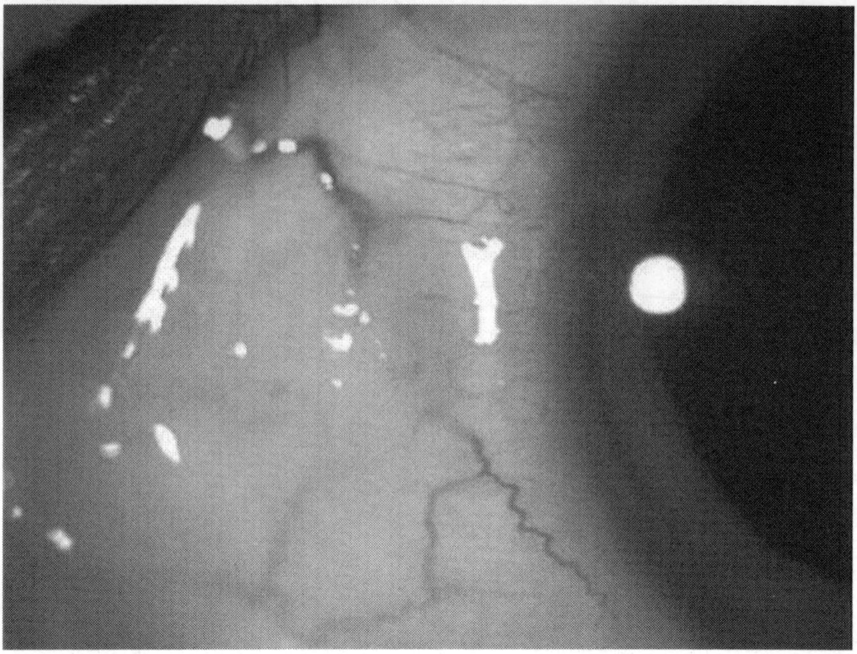

By Red eye2008 (Own work) [CC BY-SA 3.0 (http://creativecommons.org/licenses/by-sa/3.0) or GFDL (http://www.gnu.org/copyleft/fdl.html)], via Wikimedia Commons

Xanthelasma

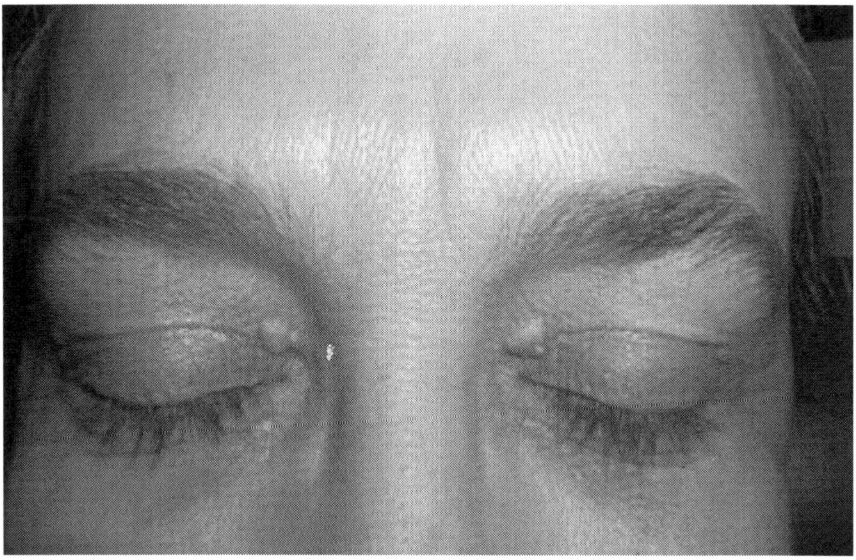

Arcus Senilis

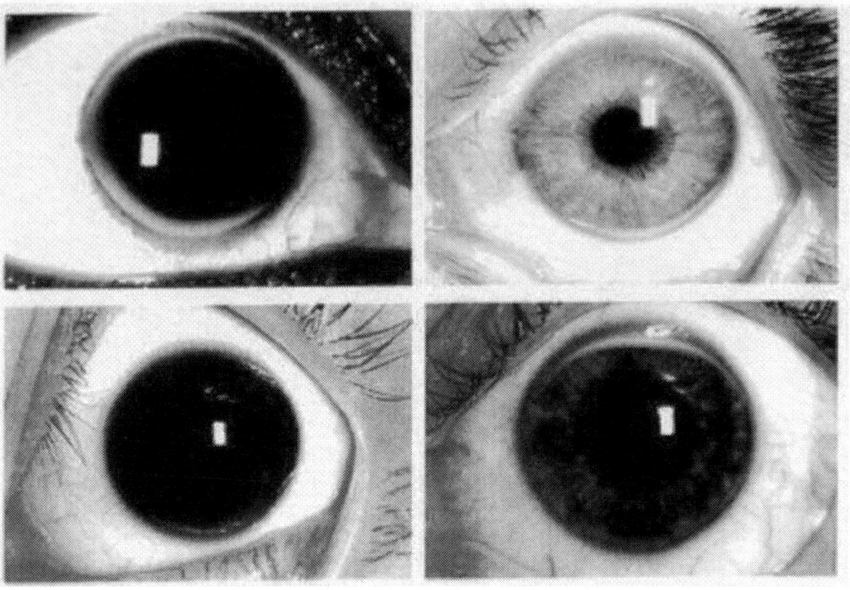

By Loren A Zech Jr and Jeffery M Hoeg [CC BY 2.0 (http://creativecommons.org/licenses/by/2.0)], via Wikimedia Commons

Ptosis

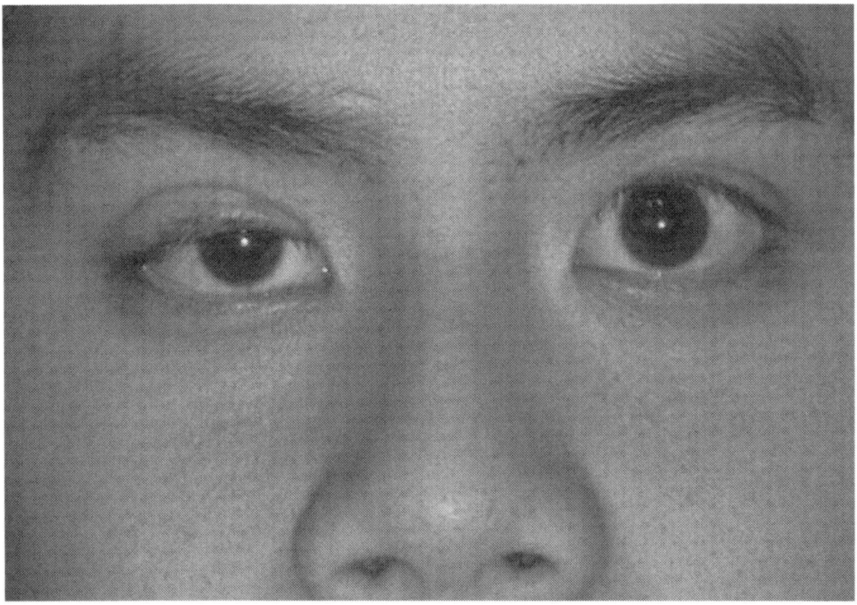

By Loren A Zech Jr and Jeffery M Hoeg [CC BY 2.0 (http://creativecommons.org/licenses/by/2.0)], via Wikimedia Commons

Exopthalmos

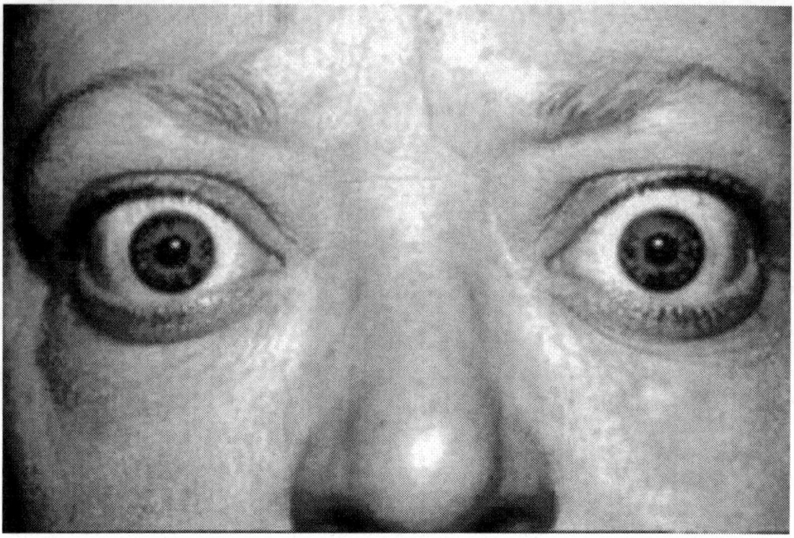

By Jonathan Trobe, M.D. - University of Michigan Kellogg Eye Center (The Eyes Have It) [CC BY 3.0 (http://creativecommons.org/licenses/by/3.0)], via Wikimedia Commons

Conjunctivitis

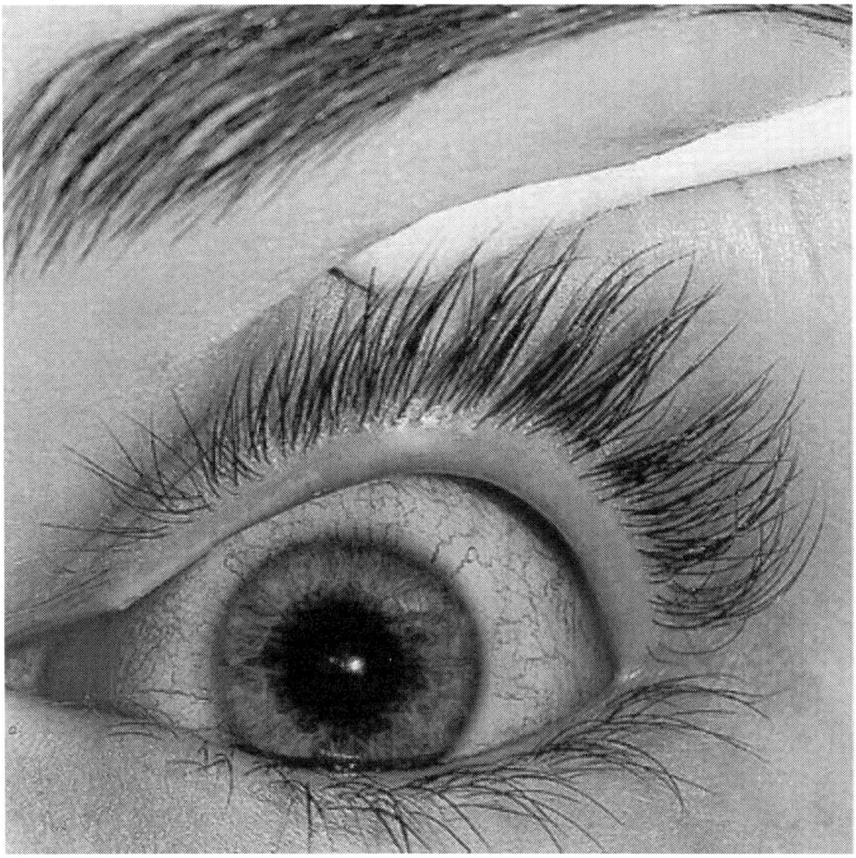

By Joyhill09 [GFDL (http://www.gnu.org/copyleft/fdl.html) or CC BY-SA 3.0 (http://creativecommons.org/licenses/by-sa/3.0)], via Wikimedia Commons

Anisocoria

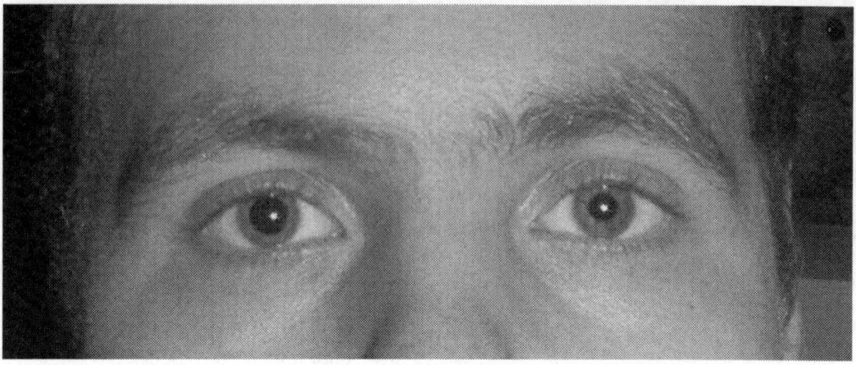

By Radomil talk (Own work) [GFDL (http://www.gnu.org/copyleft/fdl.html) or CC-BY-SA-3.0 (http://creativecommons.org/licenses/by-sa/3.0/)], via Wikimedia Commons

Miosis

By Anonymous (Anonymous) [CC0], via Wikimedia Commons

Mydriasis

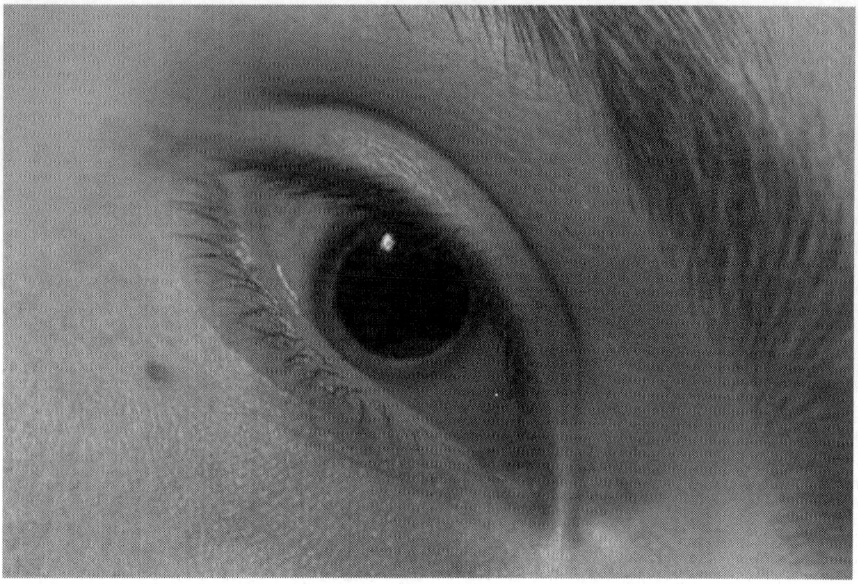

By grendel|khan and Lady Byron (Own work. Also available from my flickr.) [GFDL (http://www.gnu.org/copyleft/fdl.html), CC-BY-SA-3.0 (http://creativecommons.org/licenses/by-sa/3.0/) or CC BY-SA 2.5-2.0-1.0 (http://creativecommons.org/licenses/by-sa/2.5-2.0-1.0)], via Wikimedia Commons

Ears

Anatomy

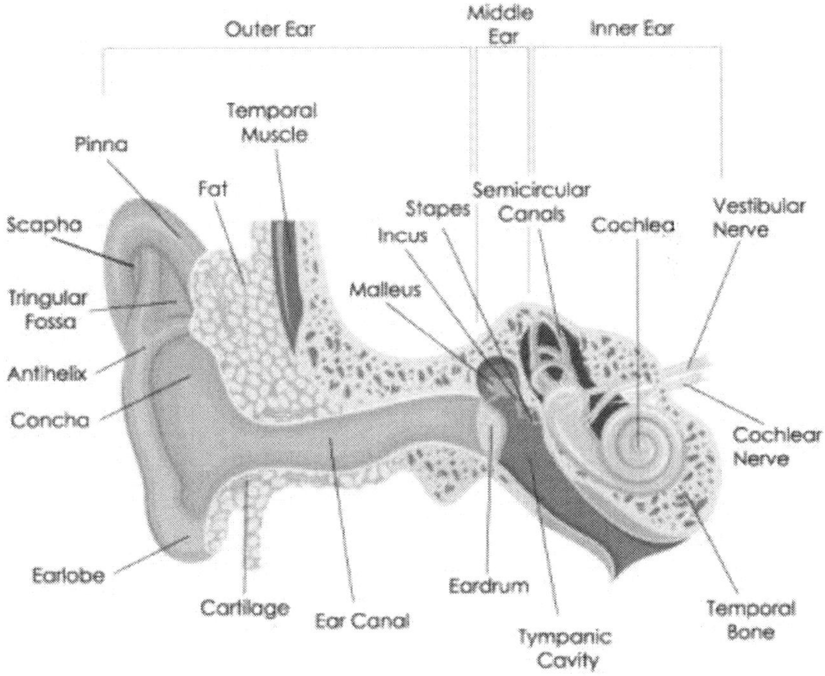

The ears are sensory organs involved with hearing and balance/equilibrium. The ear is divided in to three sections: external ear, middle ear, and inner ear.

The external ear is also known as the pinna or auricle. Sound travels into the external auditory canal and reaches the ear drum or tympanic membrane. This thin membrane separates the external and middle ear.

The ear drum vibrates in response to sound and the vibrations travel through the middle ear. The middle ear contains three small bones called ossicles: incus, malleus, and stapes.

The inner ear contains the bony labyrinth which is an opening in the temporal bone that contains the sensory organs for hearing and equilibrium.

The bony labyrinth has three parts: semicircular canals, vestibule, and cochlea. The cochlea is responsible for turning pressure from sound into impulses that communicate to the brain. The vestibular system is responsible for balance.

Inspection and Palpation

Inspect the general size and shape of the outer ear. They should be equal bilaterally with no obviously swelling or thickening. Assess skin condition, looking for lumps, lesions or tenderness. Palpating the patient's ear and mastoid process should be painless.

Inspect the external auditory meatus, there should be no swelling or redness. Most patients will have some cerumen, but excessive cerumen would be abnormal.

Inspection of the interior of the ear is called the otoscopic examination. Choose the largest speculum that fits inside the patient's ear comfortably. For adults, pull the pinna up and back. This helps straighten out the ear canal.

Hold the otoscope upside down with the dorsum of your hand along the person's cheek. Inspect the external canal, notice any redness, swelling, discharge, or any foreign bodies within the ear canal.

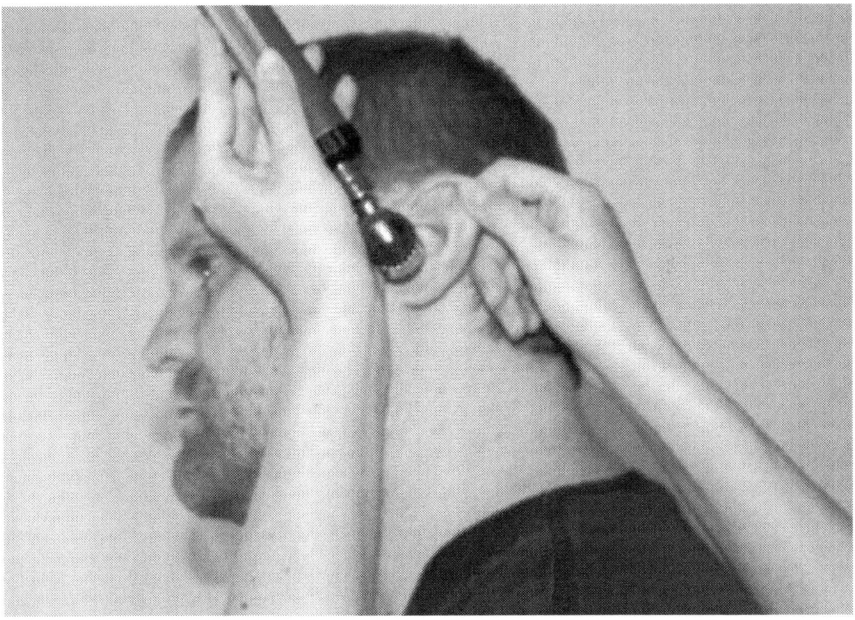

Assess the tympanic membrane by assessing the color and characteristics. It should be translucent with a pearly grey color.

The ear drum should be flat and slightly pulled in at the center. The tympanic membrane should be completely intact.

Asses hearing acuity by beginning with the whisper voice test. Stand about 2 feet away and whisper 2 syllable words into the patient's ear while asking them repeat the words they hear.

Assess air and bone conduction with turning forks. The Webber test involves striking a tuning fork and placing it midline on the patient's skull. The patient should hear the sound equally bilaterally.

The Rinne test compares air conduction versus bone conduction. Place the tuning fork midline on the patient's skull and ask them to state when they stop hearing the sound.

Abnormal Findings

Ear Drum Retraction

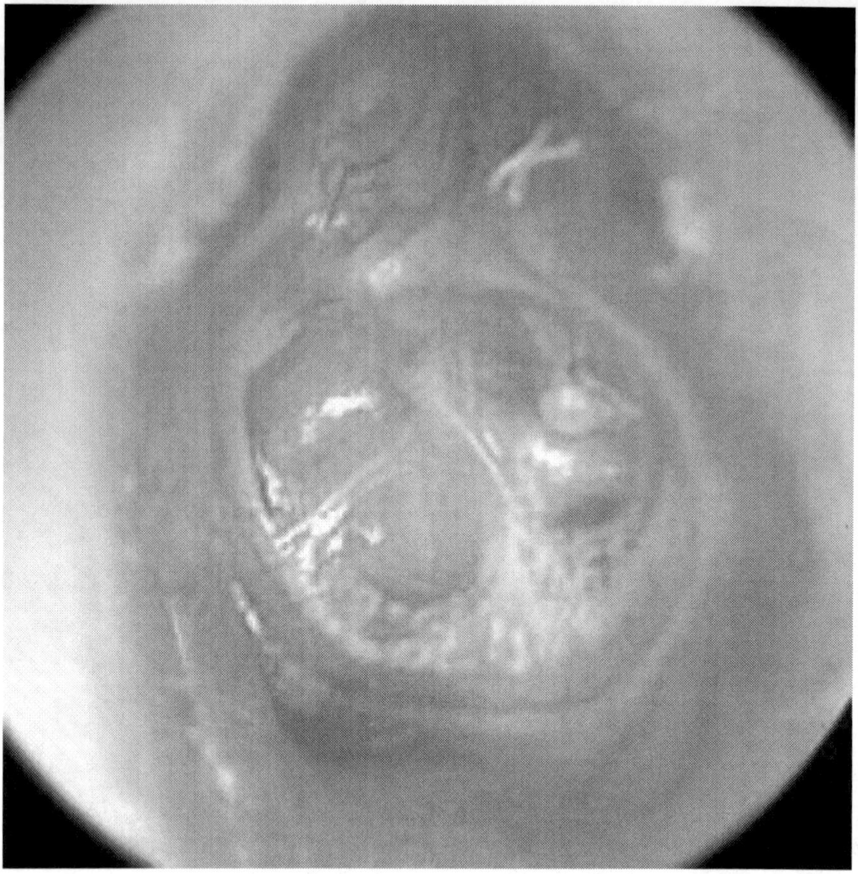

By Adrian L James (Own work) [CC BY-SA 3.0 (http://creativecommons.org/licenses/by-sa/3.0)], via Wikimedia Commons

Otitis Media

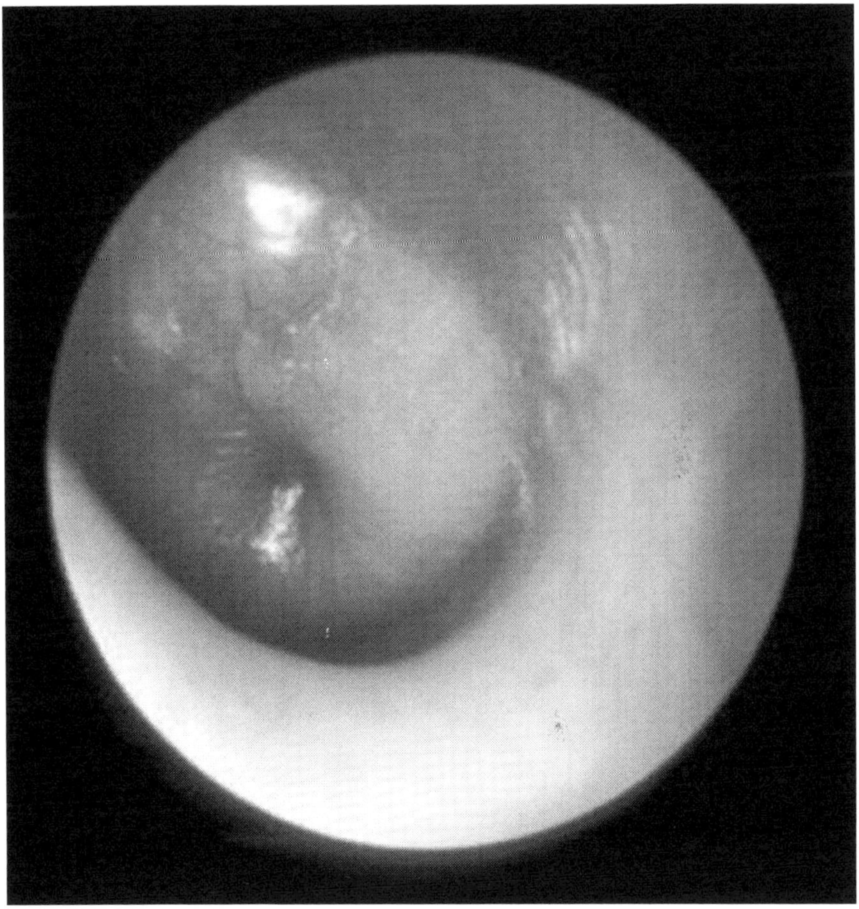

By http://www.sharinginhealth.ca (http://www.sharinginhealth.ca) [CC BY-SA 2.5 (http://creativecommons.org/licenses/by-sa/2.5)], via Wikimedia Commons

Otitis Externa

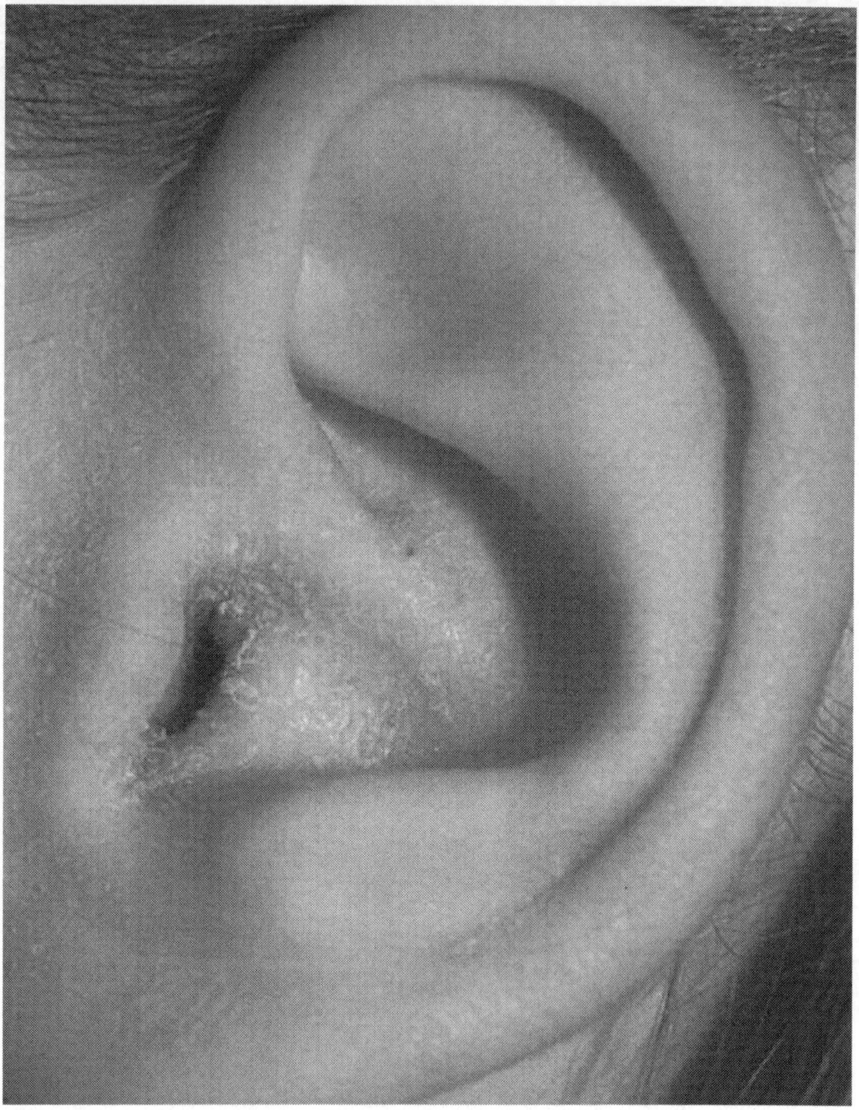

By Klaus D. Peter, Gummersbach, Germany (Own work) [CC BY 3.0 de (http://creativecommons.org/licenses/by/3.0/de/deed.en)], via Wikimedia Commons

Cauliflower Ear

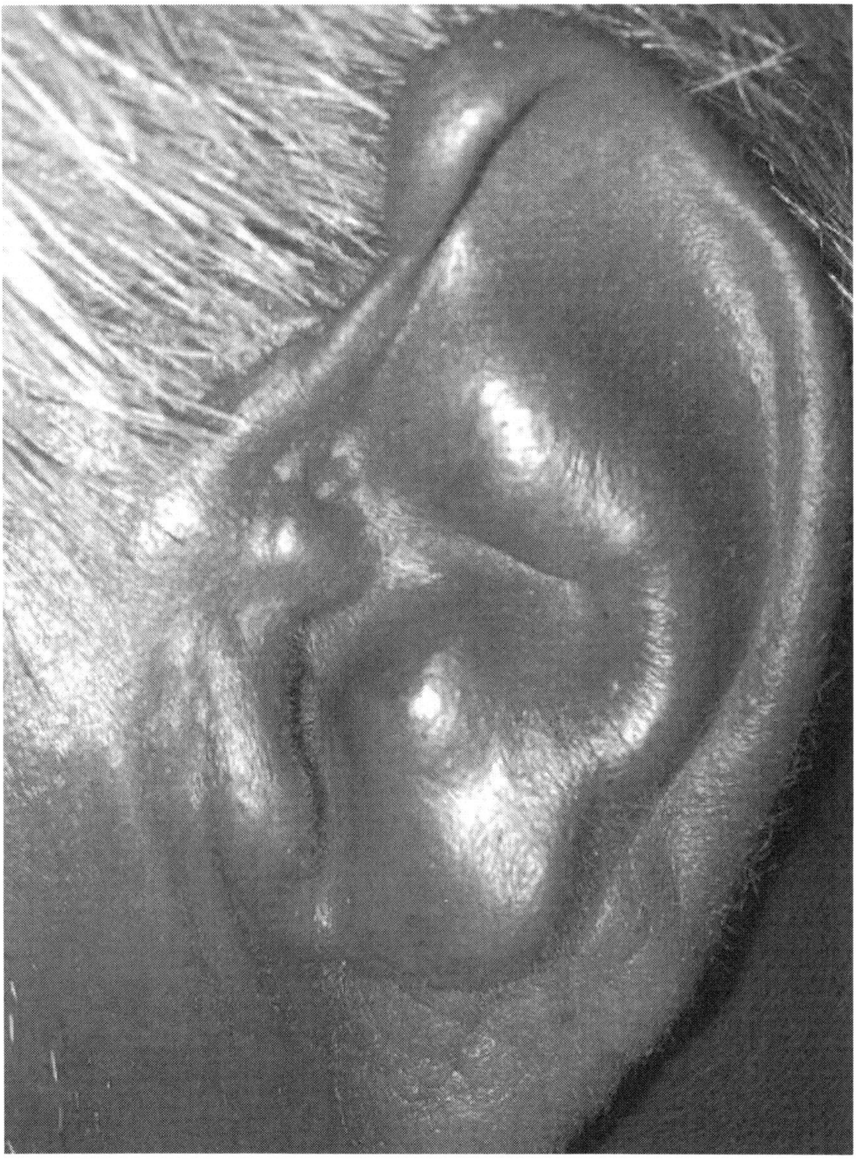

By Drvikram008 [GFDL (http://www.gnu.org/copyleft/fdl.html) or CC BY-SA 3.0 (http://creativecommons.org/licenses/by-sa/3.0)], via Wikimedia Commons

Nose

Inspection and Palpation

Inspect the nose. It should be symmetric and midline on the face. There should be no deformities or inflammation or skin lesions. Test the patency of the nostrils to reveal any obstruction in the nasal cavity.

Inspect the nasal cavity using an otoscope and a wide-tip speculum. Inspect the nasal mucosa noting its normal color and assess for any swelling or discharge.

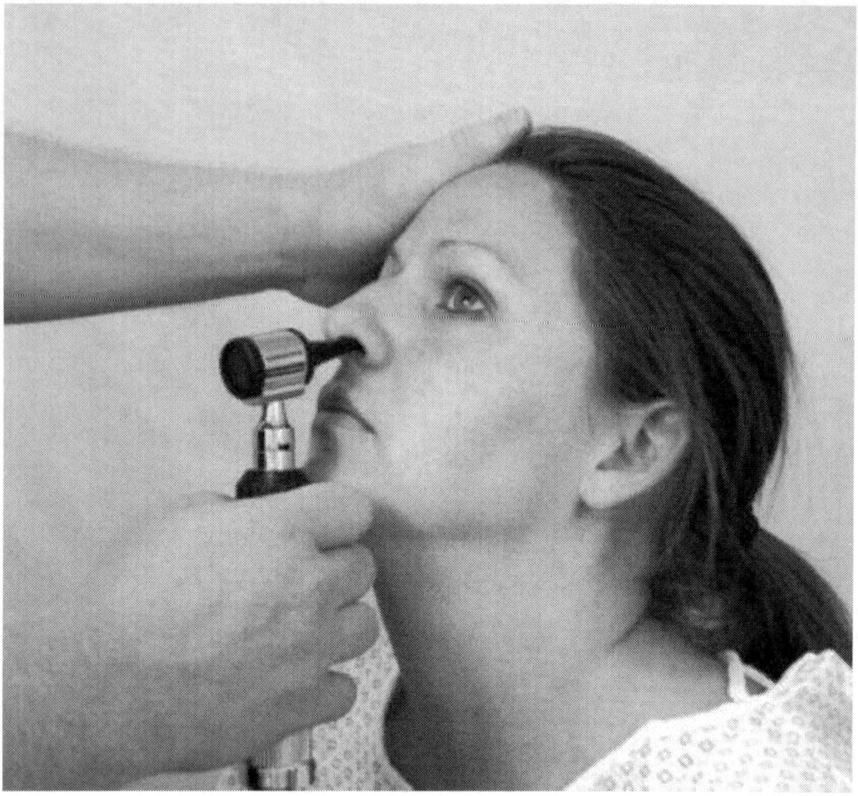

Inspect the two turbinates, the bony ridges coming down the lateral walls of the nose and also note any polyps or benign growths within the nose.

Palpate the sinus area. You should palpate the frontal sinus, which is directly below the eyebrows and the maxillary sinus right below the cheek bones. The patient will feel pressure but they should not feel pain.

Abnormal Findings

Deviated Septum

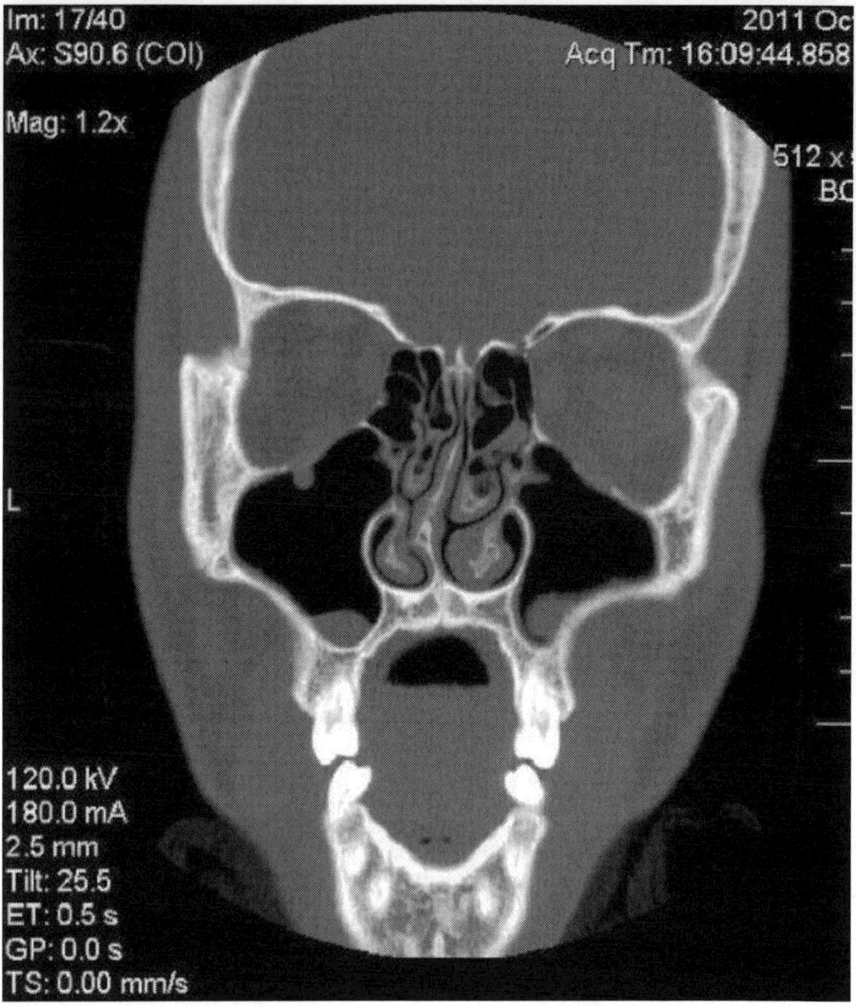

By Mike Gerkin (Own work) [CC BY-SA 3.0 (http://creativecommons.org/licenses/by-sa/3.0)], via Wikimedia Commons

Nasal Polyp

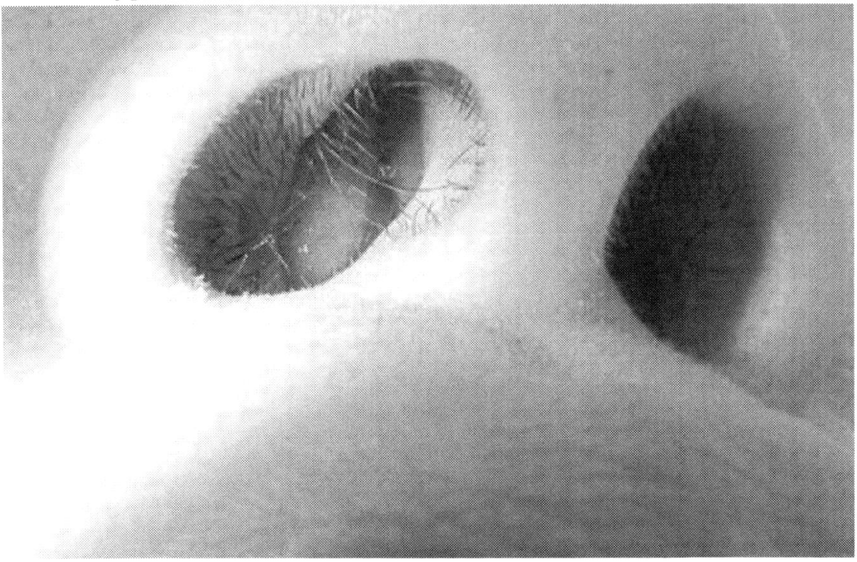

By MathieuMD (Own work) [CC BY-SA 3.0 (http://creativecommons.org/licenses/by-sa/3.0)], via Wikimedia Commons

Mouth

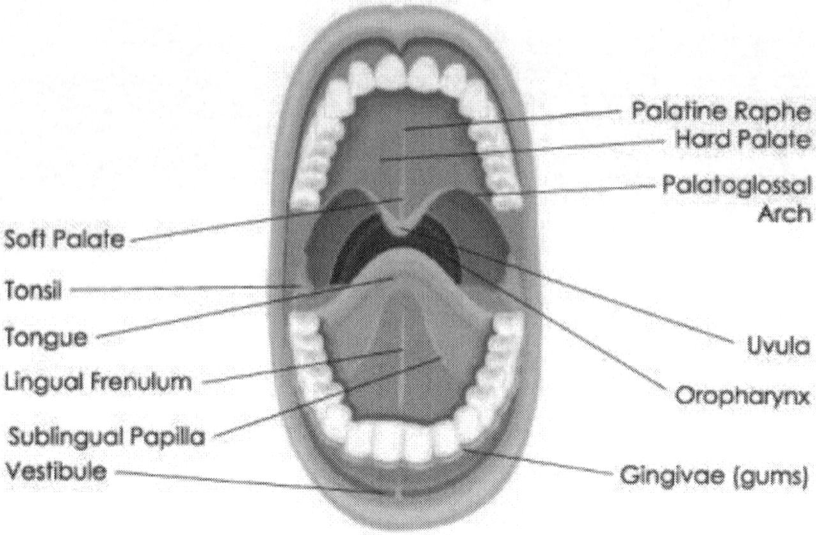

Inspection

Inspect the mouth. Inspect the lips for their color, moisture, notice any lesions or discoloration.

Inspect the teeth. The teeth should be straight and evenly spaced. There should not be any absent, loose or abnormally positioned teeth. Ask the patient to bite and note the alignment of the jaw.

Inspect the gums. The gums should look pink. Check for swelling, or any gingival margins, bleeding or discoloration.

Inspect the tongue. The tongue should be pink and symmetrical. Some patients may have a thin, white coating on their tongue.

To inspect the area beneath the tongue, have the patient touch the roof of their mouth with their tongue. Make note of any ulcerations or nodules.

Inspect the buccal mucosa, which should be soft and pink and smooth. The Stensen's duct is the opening of the parotid salivary gland.

Inspect the palate. The anterior palate is hard with rugae. The posterior palate is soft. Ask the patient to say "ah" which will cause the soft palate and the uvula to rise which aids in testing cranial nerve X, the vagus nerve.

Abnormal Findings

Cheilitis

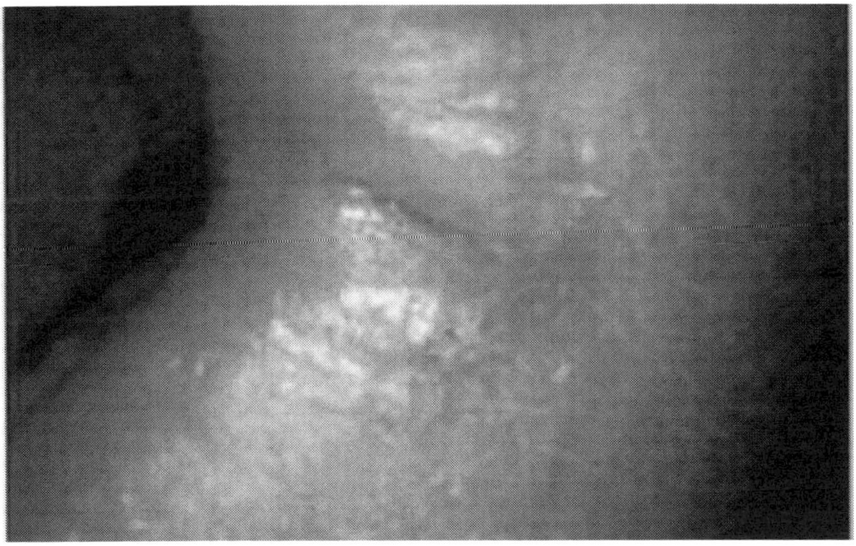

By Lesion (Own work) [CC BY-SA 3.0 (http://creativecommons.org/licenses/by-sa/3.0)], via Wikimedia Commons

Herpes

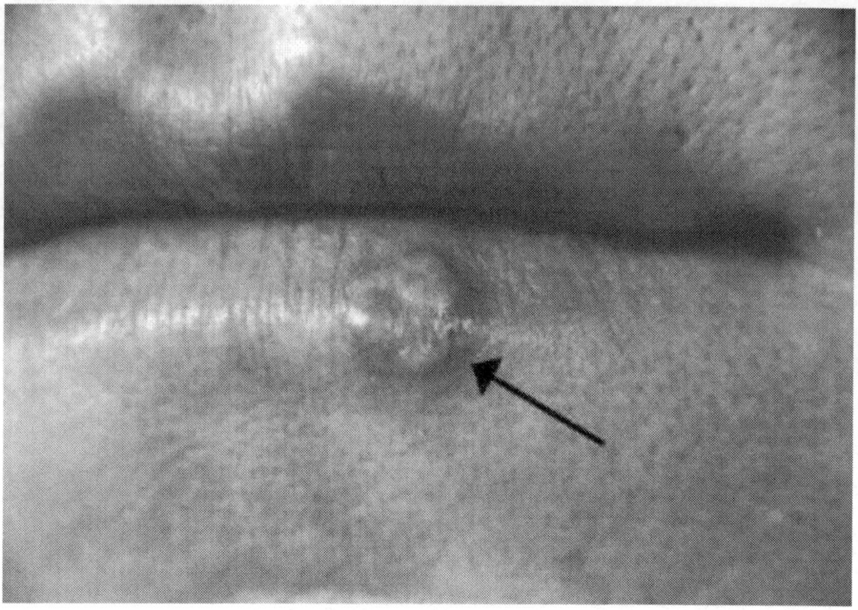

Aphthous Ulcer

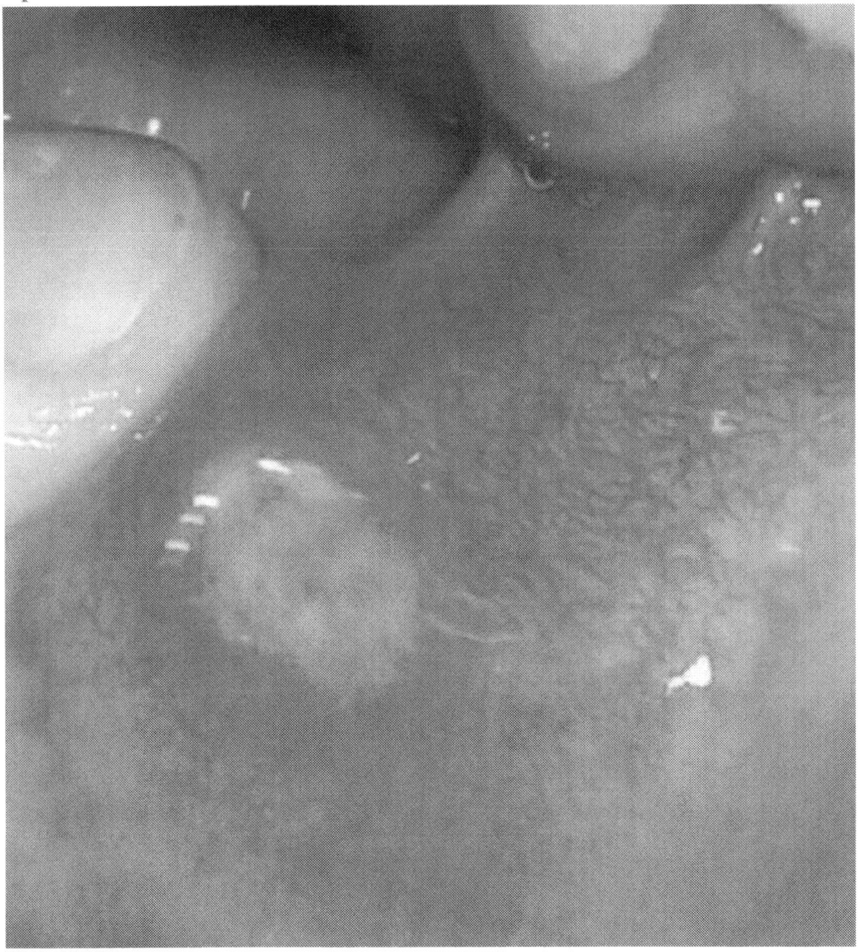

By Photographer: User:TheBlunderbuss (Own work. Published under GFDL in English Wiki) [GFDL (http://www.gnu.org/copyleft/fdl.html) or CC-BY-SA-3.0 (http://creativecommons.org/licenses/by-sa/3.0/)], via Wikimedia Commons

Torus Palantinus

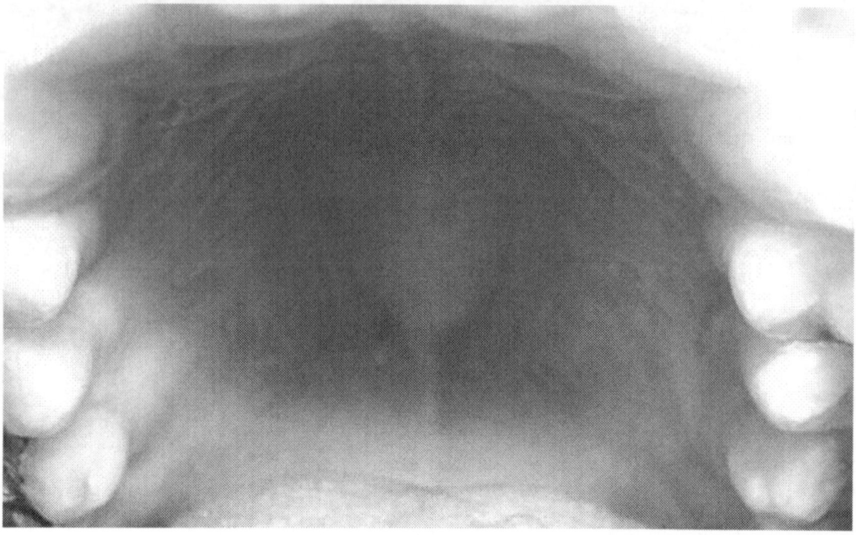

http://commons.wikimedia.org/wiki/User:Dozenist [GFDL (http://www.gnu.org/copyleft/fdl.html), CC-BY-SA-3.0 (http://creativecommons.org/licenses/by-sa/3.0/) or CC BY-SA 2.5-2.0-1.0 (http://creativecommons.org/licenses/by-sa/2.5-2.0-1.0)], via Wikimedia Commons

Throat

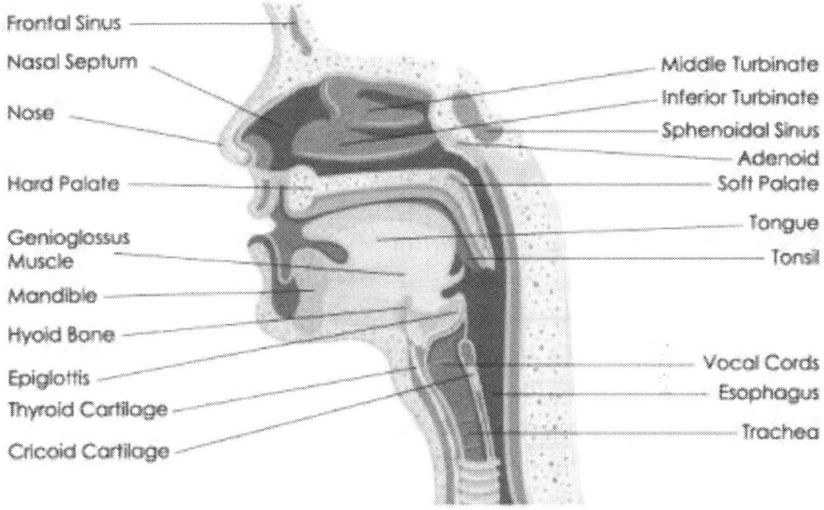

Inspection

Inspect the throat. Inspect the tonsils by having the patient open their mouth. Tonsils are graded on their size with 1+ being visible, 2+ halfway between the tonsillar pillars and uvula, 3+ touching the uvula, and 4+ touching each other. Many patients will have one plus or two plus as a normal finding.

- 1+: Visible
- 2+: Halfway between tonsillar pillars and uvula
- 3+: Touching the uvula
- 4+: Touching each other

Inspect the posterior throat for exudate or lesions. Use a tongue blade to elicit a gag reflex. Testing the gag reflex helps with assessing cranial nerves IX and X . Assess cranial nerve XII, the hypoglossal nerve, by asking the patient to stick their tongue out. The tongue should protrude midline with no deviation from side-to-side.

Abnormal Findings

Tonsillitis

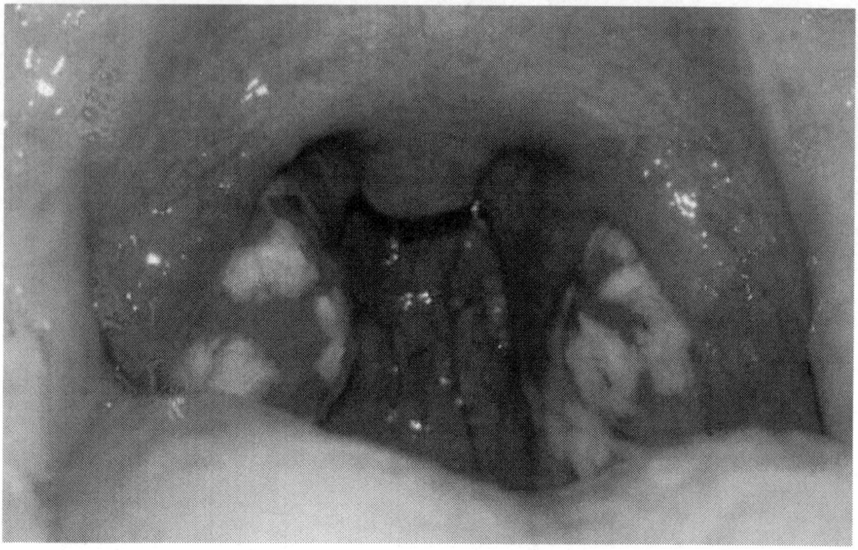

By Nick Berman (Own work) [CC BY-SA 4.0 (http://creativecommons.org/licenses/by-sa/4.0)], via Wikimedia Commons

Posterior Thorax and Lungs

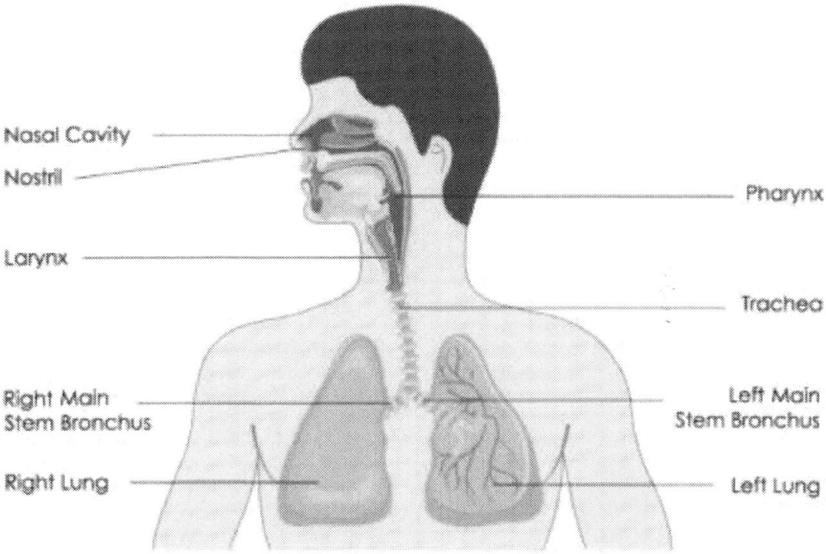

Inspection

Inspect the posterior chest, the spine, spinal process which should be straight and midline. The thorax should be symmetric. The neck and trapezius muscles should be developed normally for the age and lifestyle of the patient. The patient's skin color should be consistent with the patient's background with no abnormal coloring or lesions.

Assess the quality of the patients breathing.

Palpation

Palpate the posterior chest. Confirm symmetric chest expansion. Place your hands on the posterior chest wall between level T9 and T10. Ask the patient take a deep breath while watching your hands, they should move apart symmetrically.

Palpate for fremitus, which is a palpable vibration. This is done by placing the ball of the fingers on the patients while having them repeat the "ninety-nine".   Assess areas of the chest noting that vibration is equal corresponding areas. Fremitus will decrease as you move down.

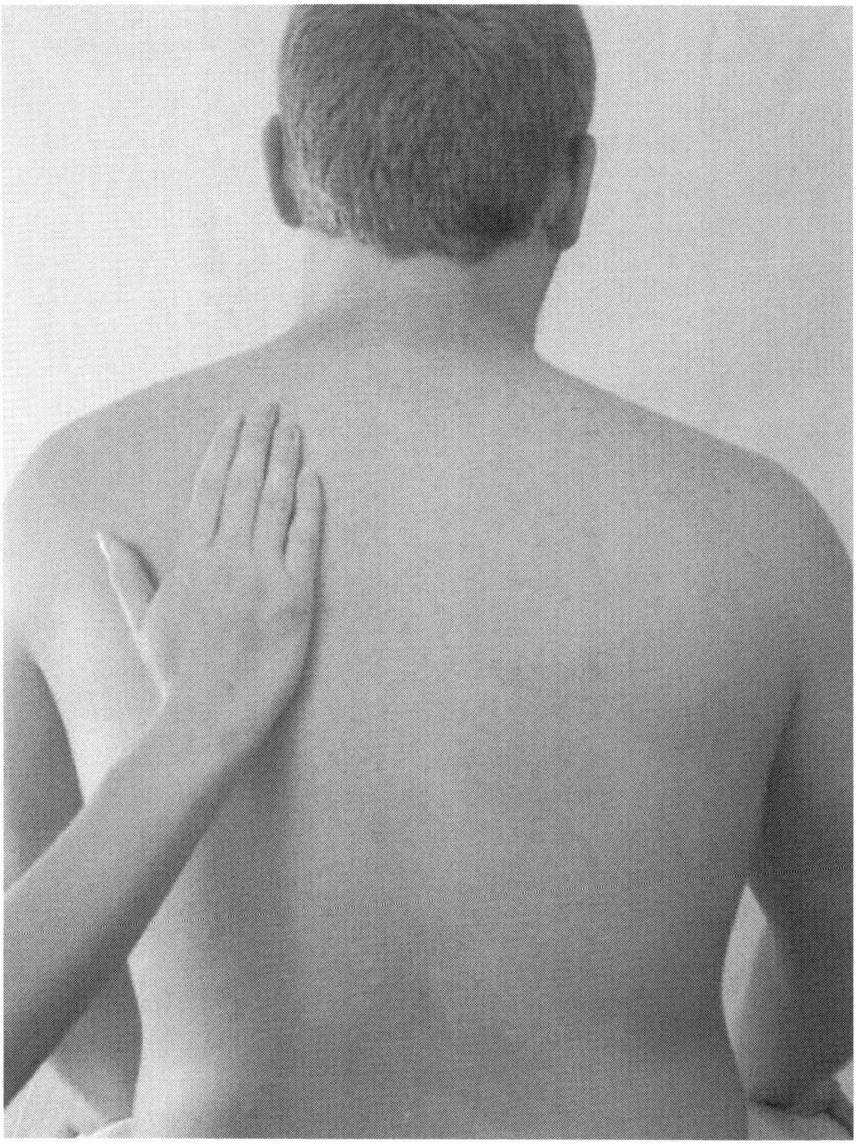

Palpate the chest wall. Notice any areas of tenderness or decreased temperature or moisture or lesions.

Percussion

Percuss of posterior chest. This is done by starting at the apex and percussing down in the intercostal spaces. Avoid bony processes like the scapula and ribs. Resonance should be heard in healthy lung tissue.

Assess diaphragmatic excursion, which is the movement of the thoracic diaphragm during breathing. This is done by percussing to map out the lower lung border during inspiration and expiration. Normal diaphragmatic excursion should be three to five centimeters.

Auscultate

Auscultate the posterior chest. Begin at the apex, around C7 and proceed to the bases around T10. Begin at C7 and move horizontally across the posterior chest. Three types of normal breast sounds whill be heard, bronchial, bronchovesicular, and vesicular. Bronchial breath sounds are high pitched and inspiration is shorter than expiration. Bronchovesicular is moderately pitched and inspiration is equal to expiration. Vesicular breath sounds are low pitched and inspiration is longer than expiration. While auscultating breath sounds, be cautious to note any adventitious breath sounds which are abnormal breath sounds.

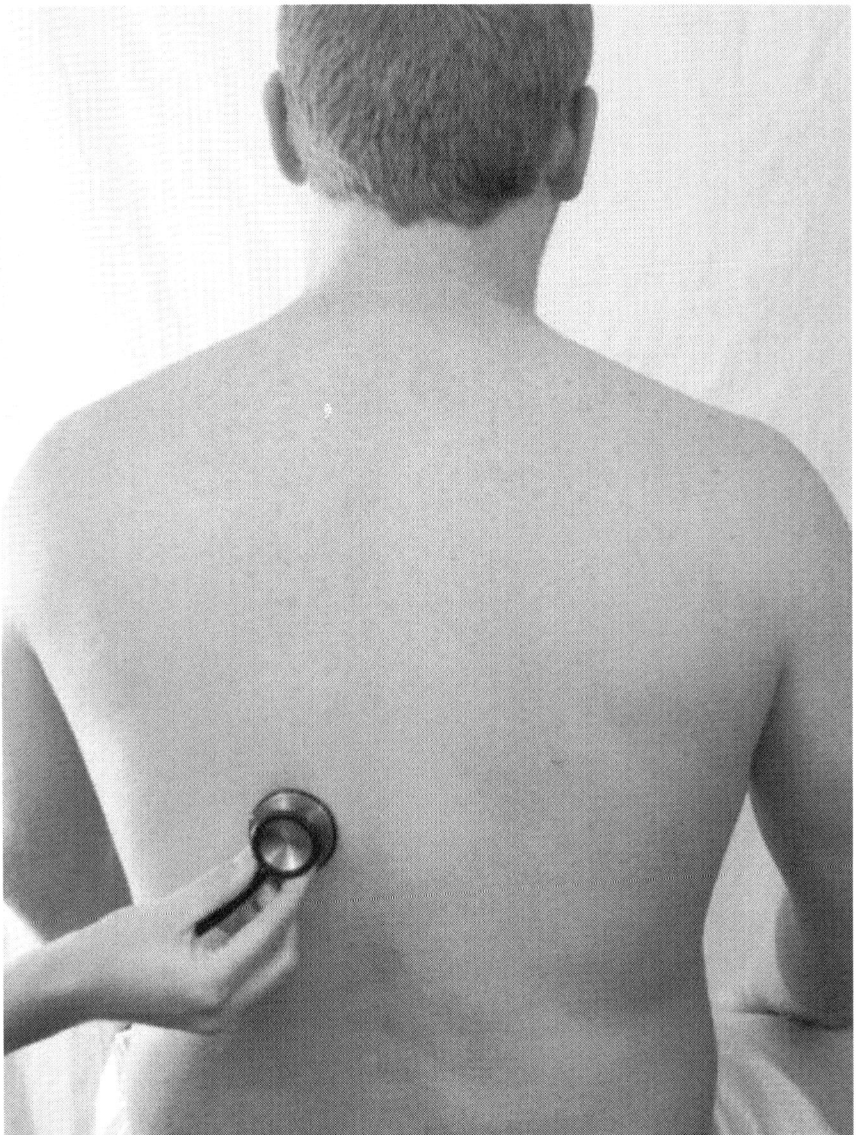

Anterior Chest

Anatomy

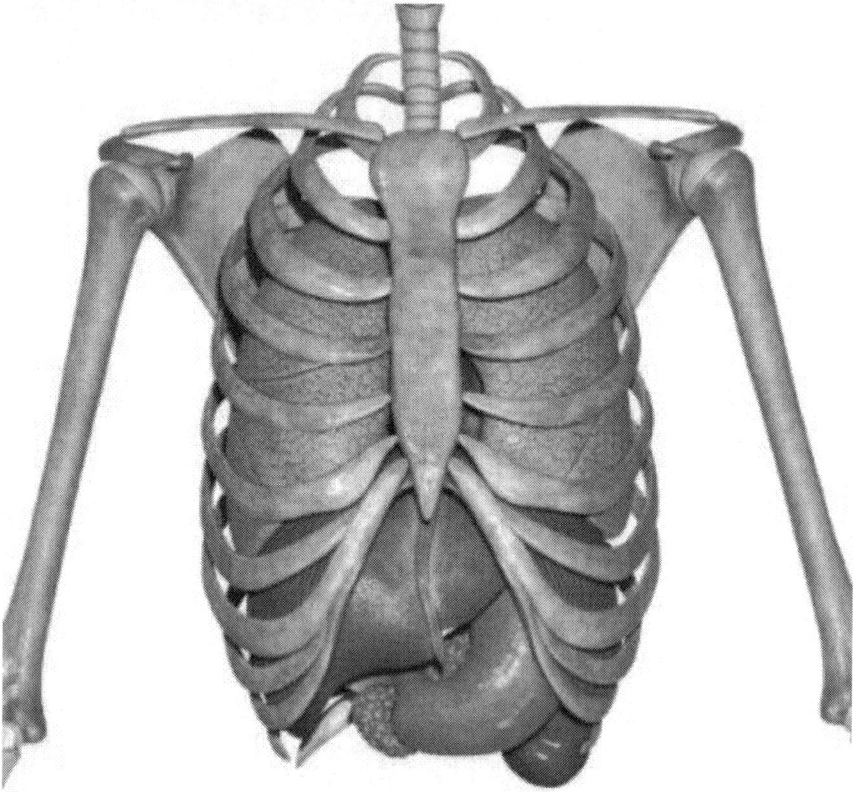

The thorax or chest refers to the area of the body between the neck and abdomen. Within the thorax is the sternum, 12 ribs and 12 thoracic vertebrae.

There are several important anatomical structures in the thorax. The suprasternal notch is a small indentation at the top of the sternum. The manubriosternal angle is where the manubrium joins to the body of the sternum. The costochondral junctions are where the ribs combine with their cartilage. The costal angle is the angle between the right and left costal margin. The zyphoid process protrudes from the bottom of the sternum this is where the right and left costal margins intersect.

The trachea begins at the cricoid cartilage in the neck and is just in front of the esophagus It splits below the sternal angle into the main bronchi. The bronchi divide into bronchioles which continue to divide. On each bronchiole are alveolar sacs filled with alveoli. The alveoli is where gas exchange occurs.

Inspection

Inspect the shape and configuration of the anterior chest noting that the ribs slope downward and are symmetric, and intercostal spaces are symmetric as well. The patients abdominal muscles should be appropriately developed for the age and activity level. The patient's face should be relaxed and they should not be showing any signs of tension.

Assess that the trachea is midline.

Assess the patient's skin color and condition and assess the quality of respirations. Normal breathing should be relaxed, regular, and effortless, and should produce no noise. Assess the patient's respiratory rate and ensure that it is within normal limits.

Percussion

Percuss the anterior chest by beginning at the apex and percussing the intercostal spaces from one side to the other in a descending motion. Dullness is heard over the heart tissue near the fifth intercostal space. In the right midclavicular line, dullness will be heard over the liver. Tympani will be evident over the gastric space.

Auscultation

Auscultate the anterior chest. This is done by beginning at the apex in the supraclavicular areas and moving down from side-to-side noting the three types of breath sounds as mentioned earlier, bronchial, bronchovesicular, and vesicular. Listen to one full respiration in each location.

Heart and Great Vessels

Anatomy

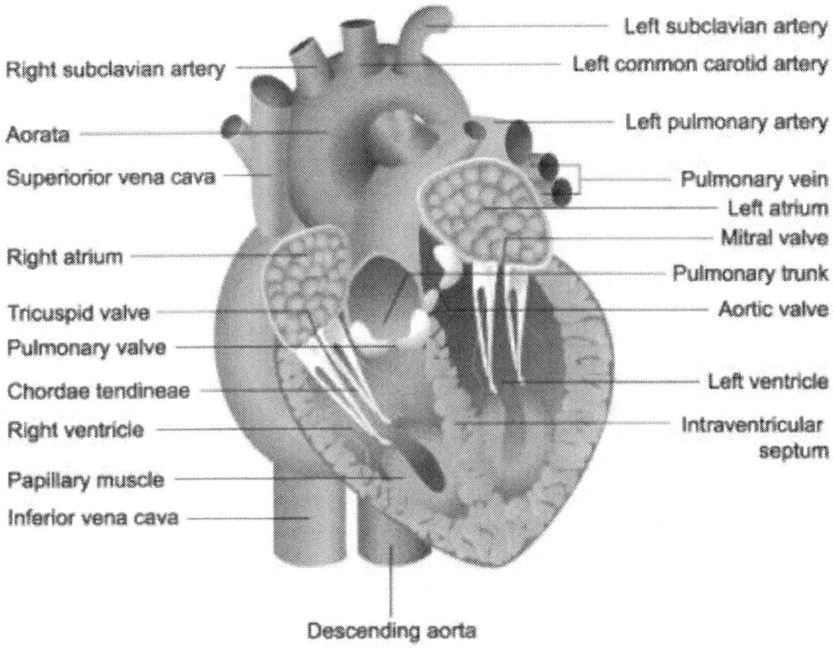

The heart is located in the chest within the rib cage from the 2nd to the 5th intercostal space and from the right side of the sternum to the midclavicular line.

The top of the heart is called the base and the bottom is the apex. The heart is divided into four chambers: right atrium and ventricle and left atrium and ventricle. The atrium holds blood while the ventricle is the strong pumping chamber.

There heart has four valves. There are two semilunar valves between the arteries and ventricles. The right is called the pulmonic valve and the left is called the aortic valve. There are two atrioventricular valves between the atria and ventricles. The right is called the tricuspid valve and the left is called the bicuspid or mitral valve. The atrioventricular valves open during diastole (relaxation while the heart is filling with blood). The seminlunar valves open during systole (during contraction so blood can be pumped out of the heart).

Heart Sounds

S1: closure of the AV valves which is the beginning of systole

S2: closure of the SL valves which is the end of systole

Inspection and Palpation

Palpate the carotid artery. Palpate one artery at a time to avoid compressing blood flow to the brain. Palpate for pulse strength and equality bilaterally.

Auscultate the carotid artery. This is especially indicated in older individuals and those who demonstrate signs of cardiovascular disease. Auscultate for bruit. Listen with the bell of the stethoscope and apply over one carotid artery at a time being cautious not to apply any direct pressure to avoid creating an artificial bruit.

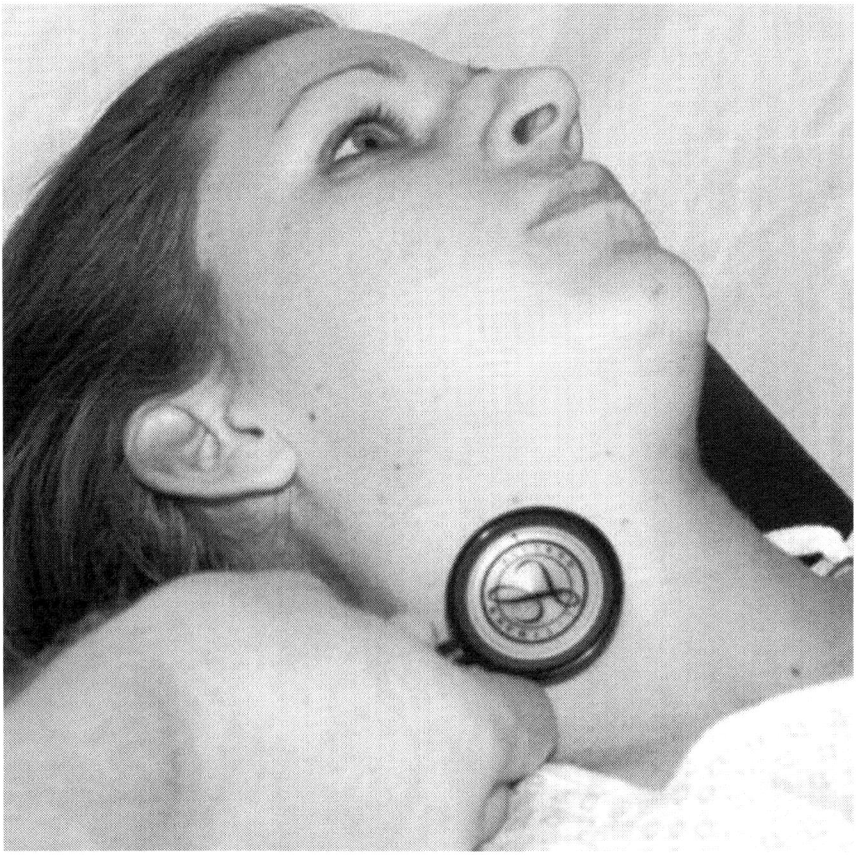

Inspect the jugular venous pulse. This is done by laying the patient at an angle from 30 to 45 degrees to avoid flexing the neck. Ask the patient to turn their head away from the examiner while shining a bright light on the neck. This will highlight the pulsation and shadows of the jugular venous pulse. As a person is raised to the sitting position, the jugular should flatten and disappear usually around 45 degrees.

Inspect the anterior chest for a visible apical impulse. This is also known as point of maximum impulse. If visible, this should be over the fifth intercostal space.

Palpate the apical pulse. This can be done with just one finger pad. Note the location, which should be over the fifth intercostal space, the size, amplitude, and duration. The apical pulse may not be palpable with many patients.

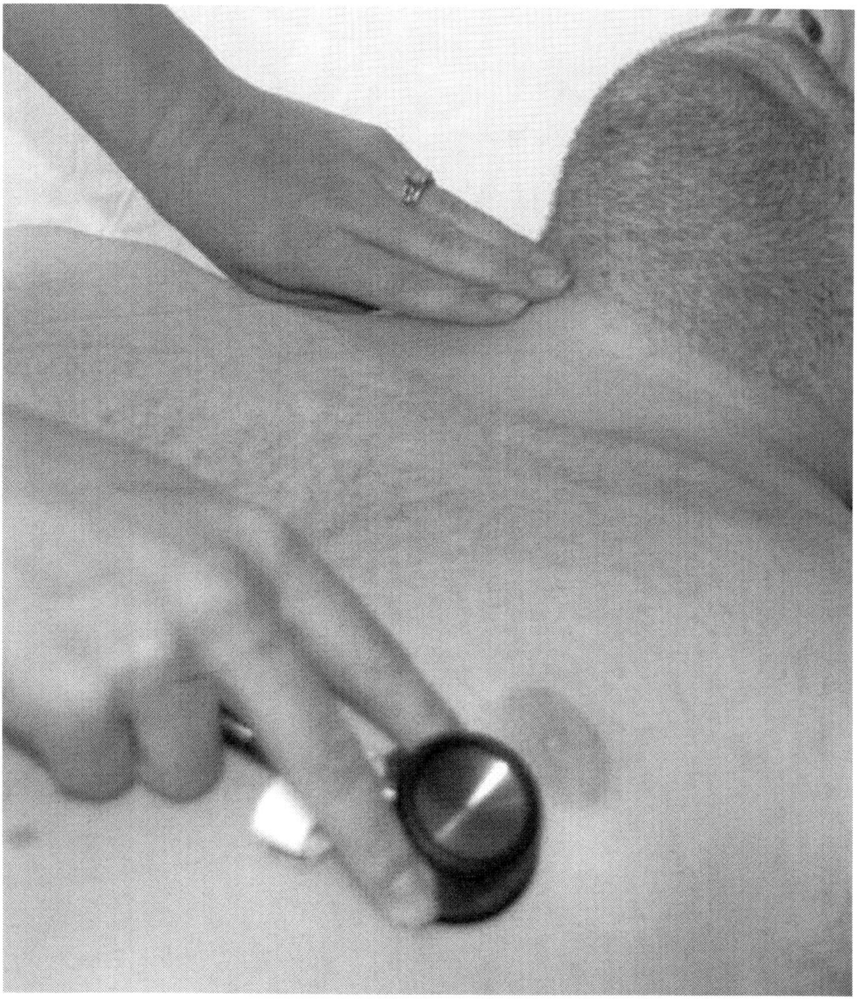

Palpate across the precordium. With the palms of four fingers palpate gently across the precordium assessing for any other pulsations.

Auscultate

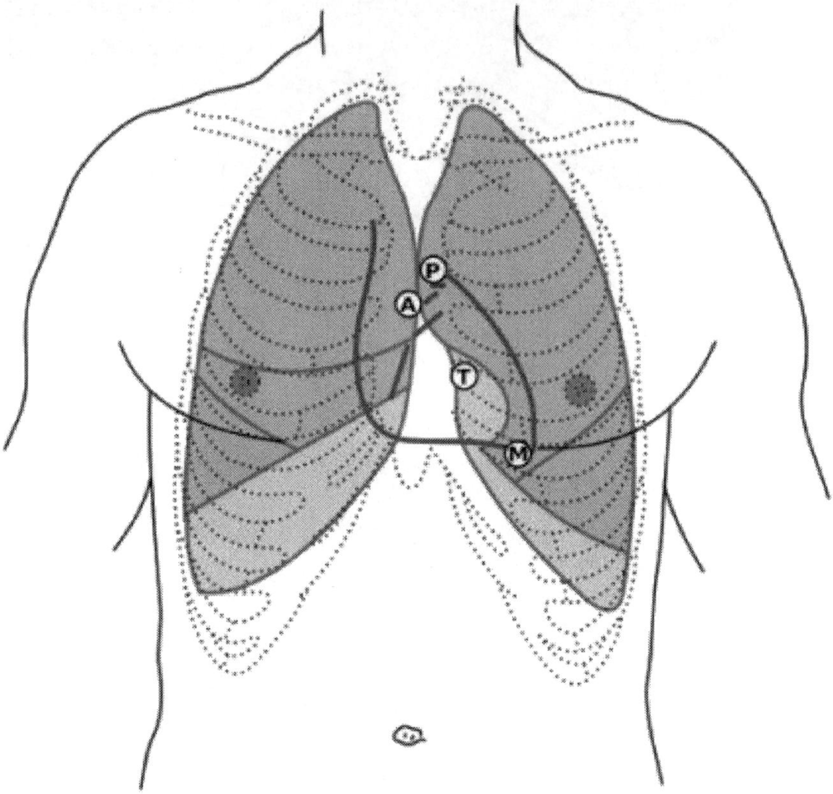

By Madhero88 (Own work Reference netter image) [CC BY-SA 3.0 (http://creativecommons.org/licenses/by-sa/3.0)], via Wikimedia Commons

Auscultate the heart sounds. Auscultate the four valve areas. These auscultation areas are not over the anatomical structures, but rather over the areas where sounds are most pronounced and most easily heard. The mnemonic APE To Man is useful in recalling the order of auscultation. APE would stand for aortic, pulmonic, and Erb's point; To Man, tricuspid and mitral.

The aortic valve should be located over the second right intercostal space. The pulmonic valve auscultation area should be located over the second left intercostal space. The tricuspid valve area would be over the left lower sternal border and the mitral valve can be heard over the fifth intercostal space around the left midclavicular line. Actual locations of heart sounds may vary from patient to patient.

Auscultate with the bell for murmurs. Auscultate for any S3 and S4 murmur sounds. Note the rhythm of the heart and the rate. Listen to S1 and S2 separately and listen for any sorts of splitting or murmurs. Murmurs are classified by their timing, loudness which is graded from grade one through six. The pitch and the pattern, the quality, location, radiation, posture.

Peripheral Vascular System

Anatomy

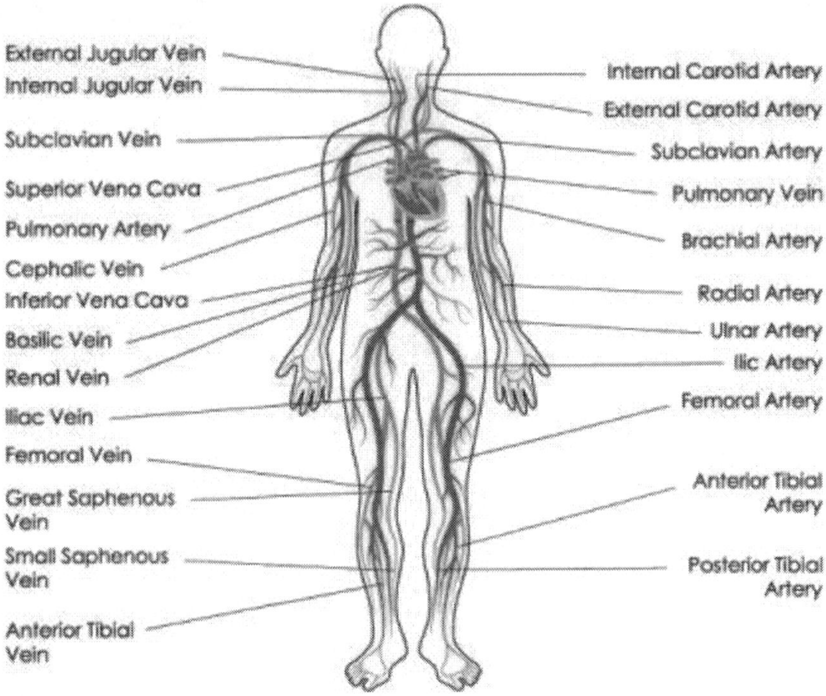

The peripheral vascular system is the transport system in the body. Vessels in the body contain fluids which can carry a variety of substances throughout the body. The heart pumps blood to the lungs where blood picks up oxygen and returns the heart.

The heart then deliveries the oxygenated blood and nutrients to the body via arteries. Once oxygen has been picked up by cells in the body blood and waste travels back the heart via veins.

Inspection and Palpation

Inspect and palpate the arms. Note the color of the skin and the nail beds, the temperature, texture, turgor of the skin and assess for any lesions and edema.

Assess capillary refill. This is done by depressing the nail beds and assessing how long it takes for the color to return. This should happen within one to two seconds.

The arms should be symmetric in size. Assess pulses in all extremities. Palpate radial pulses and dorsalis pedis pulses. Normal would be +2 pulse and they are graded from 0-+3.

Inspect and palpate the legs. Inspect color, hair growth, venous pattern, any swelling or lesions. Inspect the hair to see if hair growth is even throughout the legs.

Legs should be symmetric in size without new swelling or atrophy. Assess calf circumference and measure the widest part in exactly the same on either side.

Palpate to assess the temperature. Palpate the inguinal lymph nodes and note for any unusual size and make sure that they are non-tender.

Palpate peripheral arteries in both legs. The femoral pulse is found just below the inguinal ligament halfway between the pubis and the anterior-superior iliac spine. Palpate popliteal pulses. This is done with the person's leg extended and relaxed with the examiners fingers just underneath. Posterior tibial pulses are found along the medial malleolus. The dorsalis pedis pulse is lateral and parallel to the big toe.

Doppler may be required to assess these pulses if they are not easily palpated. If doppler is required, mark the location of the pulse with a marker.

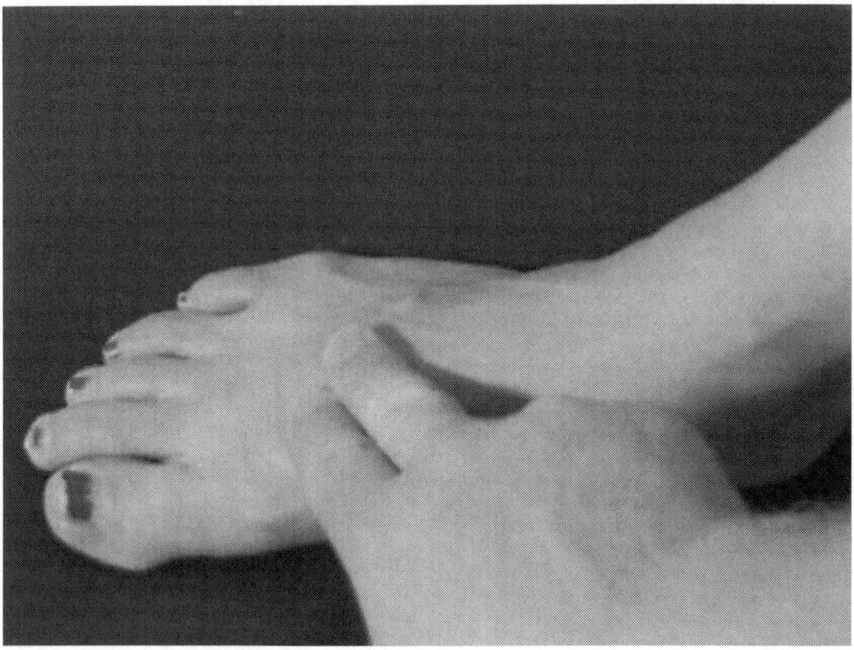

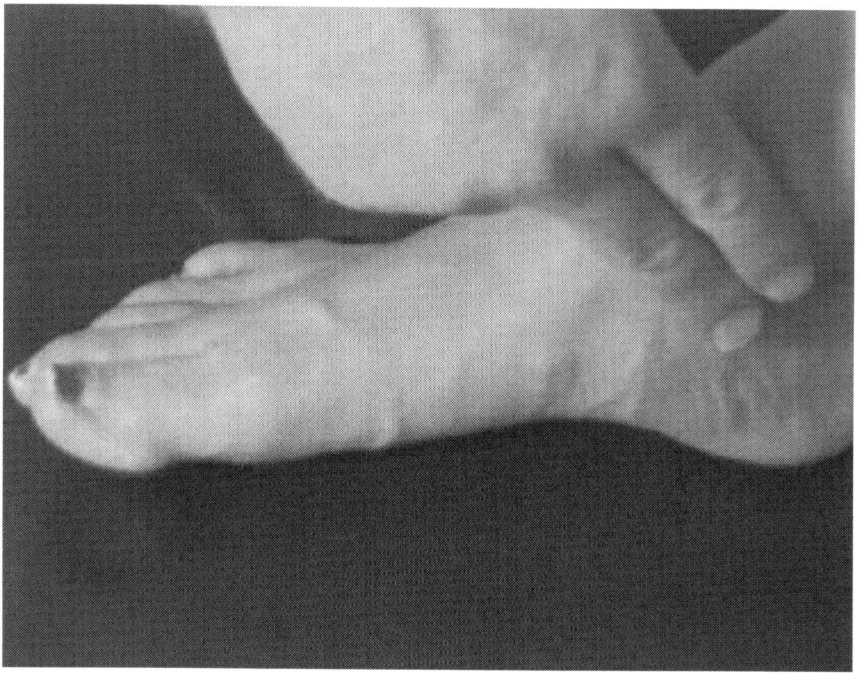

Assess for peripheral edema. Edema is graded from 1+ to 4+.

- 1+: being mild pitting and no swelling of the leg
- 2+: moderate: both feet plus lower legs, hands or lower arms
- 3+: severe: generalized bilateral pitting edema, both feet legs, arms, and face
- 4+: very deep pitting and indentation lasts a long time and the leg appears to be very swollen

Abnormal Findings

Peripheral Artery Disease (Arterial Ulcer)

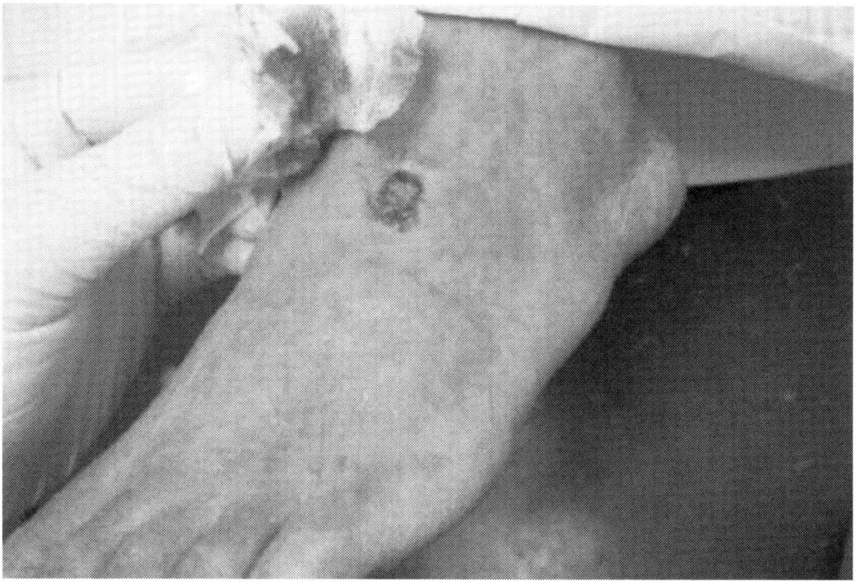

By Jonathan Moore [CC BY 3.0 (http://creativecommons.org/licenses/by/3.0)], via Wikimedia Commons

Chronic Venous Insufficiency

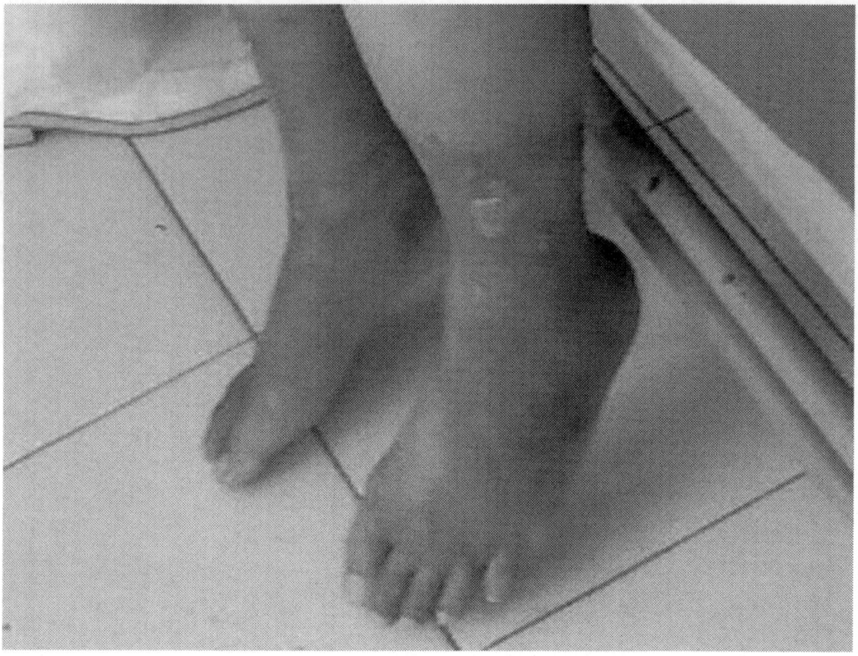

Pitting Edema

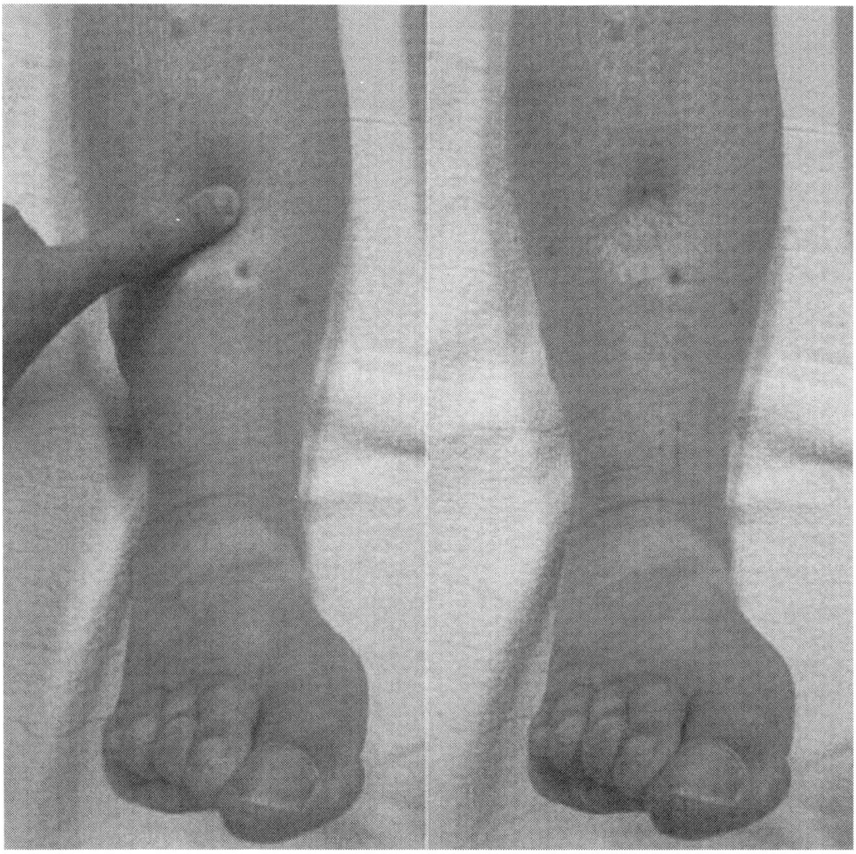

Abdomen

Anatomy

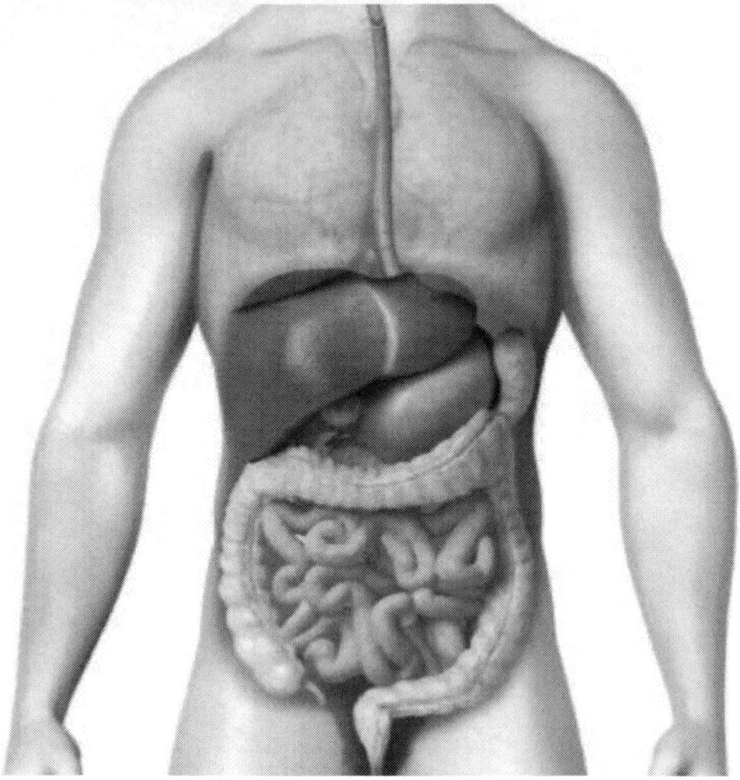

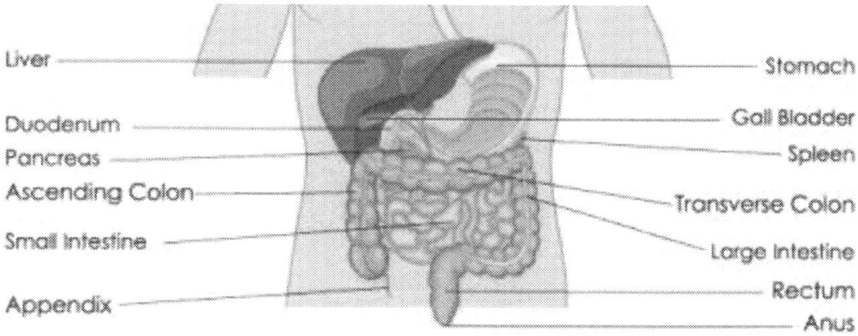

The abdomen is a large cavity below the diaphragm. The largest artery in the abdomen is the aorta which splits into the iliac arteries. The inferior vena cava runs parallel to the aorta and splits into two iliac veins. Within the abdomen the liver, pancreas, stomach, appendix, spleen, gallbladder, kidneys, intestines, colon, and reproductive organs are located.

Pancreas: The pancreas is located in the abdomen behind the stomach. It has endocrine functions and exocrine functions. Then pancreas produces important hormones like insulin and glucagon. The pancreas also produces enzymes that help with digestion and absorption of food in the intestines.

Appendix: The appendix is located right where the small intestines join the large intestines. The function of the appendix is unknown, but it can often become inflamed and can sometimes burst.

Stomach: The stomach is an important part of the digestive system. It is located in the upper left quadrant of the abdomen. Food enters the stomach from the esophagus through the lower esophageal sphincter. It mixes with proteases (which breakdown protein) and hydrochloric acid. The stomach muscles thoroughly mix the food to help break it down. Food leaves the stomach through the pyloric sphincter into the intestines.

Spleen: The spleen is located in the abdomen just left of the stomach. The spleen helps remove old red blood cells and hold a store of blood. It also synthesizes antibodies.

Small intestines: Once food has been mixed in the stomach the contents, called chyme then move into the duodenum of the small intestine. Secretin stimulates release of bicarbonate which helps neutralize the acidity of the chyme. Bile from the gallbladder helps emulsify fats and enzymes from the pancreas help breakdown carbohydrate, fat, and protein. Iron is absorbed in the duodenum. The food then moves into the jejunum where most nutrients are absorbed into the blood stream. The final segment of the intestines is called the ileum. Vitamin B12 and bile salts are absorbed in the ileum. The intestines contains many small projections called villi that significantly increase surface area for absorption of nutrients.

Large intestines: Waste that isn't absorbed in the intestines then travels through the segments of the colon: ascending colon, transverse colon, descending colon, sigmoid colon. Water is reabsorbed in the colon. Waste then travels through the rectosigmoid junction into the rectum and is excreted via the anal canal.

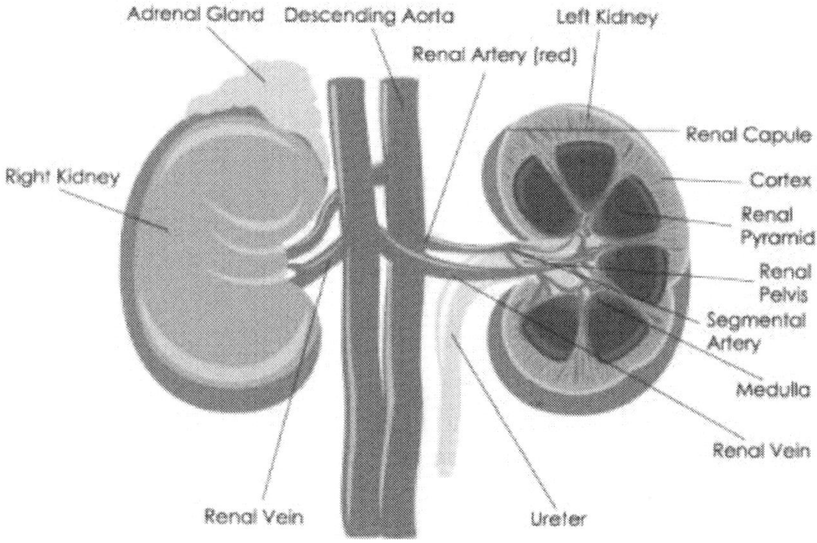

Kidney: There are two kidneys in the body. They lie on the right and left side of abdomen below the liver and stomach respectively. They sit toward the back of the abdomen. An adrenal gland sits directly above each bean shaped kidney. A renal artery enters the kidney and the renal vein and ureter exit the kidney. The functional unit of the kidney is the nephron. The nephron helps filter out excess water and solutes from the blood. Filtered blood then leaves via the renal vein, and waste via the ureter.

The kidneys play many vital roles in the body including removal of waste products; regulation of blood pressure and electrolytes; acid-base balance; reabsorption of amino acids, glucose, and water; hormone production: calcitriol, erythropoietin; and enzyme production: renin.

Liver: The liver is located in the upper right quadrant of the abdomen. The liver has two lobes and sits protected below the ribs Once blood has picked up nutrients from the intestines its first stop is the liver. The liver removes chemicals and breaks down drugs.

The liver produces bile which is secreted into the intestines to aid in the absorption of fat. It can synthesize, glucose, amino acids, proteins, cholesterol, and triglycerides, and produce clotting factors. The liver stores glycogen (carbohydrate) and fat soluble vitamins, converts ammonia into urea, and conjugates bilirubin for excretion. This is not an all inclusive list, just an overview of some of the liver's most important functions.

Gallbladder: The Gallbladder is located under the liver. Once the liver produces bile it travels to the gallbladder for storage. When a meal is ingested the gallbladder can release the stored bile into the intestines to aid in the absorption of fats.

Inspection

Inspect the contour of the abdomen. This is done by stooping to view across the abdomen to determine if it is flat to slightly rounded. Assess the symmetry of the abdomen by shining a light across and assessing for any bulging or visible masses, or asymmetry.

Assess the umbilicus, and notice any discoloration, inflammation or hernia. There should be none.

Assess the skin texture and color. There should be no lesions or scars. If scars are present note the length and general nature.

Assess for any pulsations or movement in the abdominal area. In some individuals, it may be possible to see pulsations of the aorta. Respiratory movements may also be seen in patients.

Peristalsis may be visible in some patients.

Auscultate

Auscultation comes after inspection in the abdomen so that palpation does not disrupt bowel sounds and change your assessment.

Begin in the right lower quadrant, and use the diaphragm of the stethoscope pressed lightly against the skin. Note bowel sound characteristics and frequency. They should be anywhere from five to 30 times per minute.

It is not necessary to count bowel sounds, but note if they are hypoactive, hyperactive or normal. Listen for one full minute in each abdominal quadrant to determine activity.

Auscultate vascular sounds within the abdomen. You should listen for any bruits, and you're going to be listening to the aorta, the left renal artery, the iliac artery and the femoral artery. You may need to use firmer pressure to listen for these sounds.

Percussion

Percuss for tympany. Percuss to determine the location and size of the liver and the spleen. Percuss in all four quadrants. Tympany will be heard due to air in the intestines. A duller sound would indicate a mass, or distended bladder, or adipose tissue.

To measure the size of the liver, begin in the right midclavicular line. Percuss down the right midclavicular line, listening for when lung resonance stops, the sound will change to a dull sound. Mark that spot, which should be around the fifth intercostal space. Continue percussion until tympany is heard once again. This indicates the lower border of the liver.

Measure the distance between the two marks. This indicates the size of the liver. It should range from 6 to 12 centimeters in healthy adults.

To assess the spleen begin by percussing a dull tone over the ninth to eleventh intercostal space, on the left midaxillary line.

Percussion of the kidneys aids in assessment of pain and tenderness. This is done by placing the nondominant hand over the costovertebral angle. The nondominant hand is struck with the ulnar surface of the dominate hand made into a fist. Repeat over both kidneys.

Palpation

Begin palpation by working from light to deep palpation. You begin with light palpation with the forefingers close together, and you should make a small circular motion. Lift the fingers between the quadrants. As you're moving around the patient, you should assess for any guarding and notice if the patient is feeling pain.

Upon completion of light palpation move on to deep palpation. To do this place two hands, one on top of the other, the top hand pushes the bottom hand. As this is done, take note of the location size and consistency of the abdomen, as well as any tenderness.

Assess for the colon, there may be some tenderness over the colon which is a normal finding. If a mass is felt note the location, size, consistency, and any tenderness.

Assess the location of the liver, via palpation. Place your left hand under the person's back, and lift up to support the abdominal contents. You should then place your right hand on the right upper quadrant, and push deeply down and under the right costal margin. The person should take a deep breath, and with this you should be able to feel the edge of the liver. The liver may not be palpable.

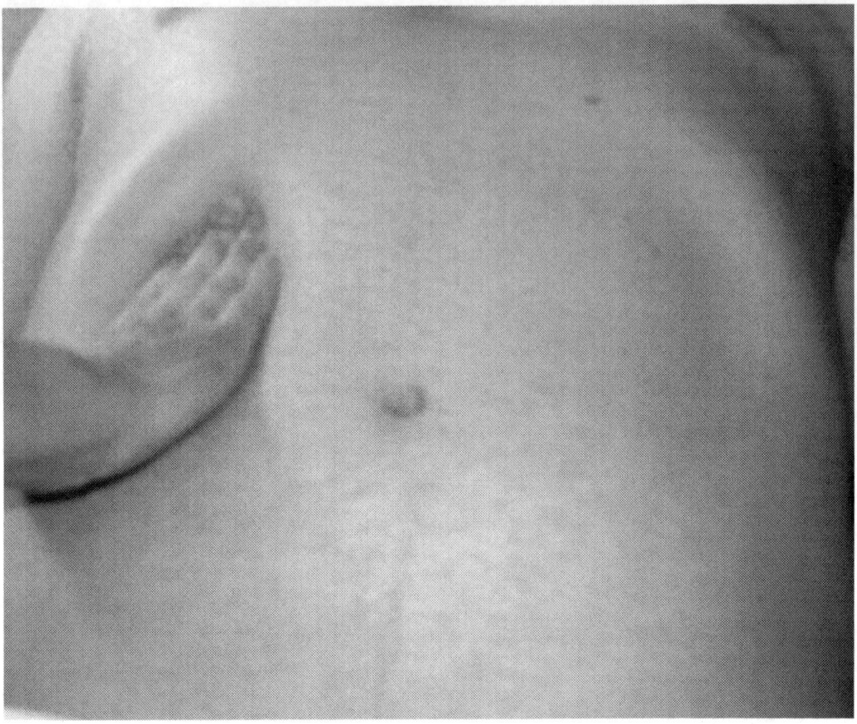

The spleen generally is not palpable. If it is palpable, it may be due to being enlarged. Reach your left hand over the abdomen, and behind the left side of the eleventh and twelfth ribs. You should then place your right hand on the left upper quadrant, with the right fingers pointing towards the left axilla. Push your hand deeply down under the left costal margin. Ask the person to take a deep breath.

When assessing the kidneys place your hands together and position them at the person's right flank, and then press firmly and deeply, and ask the person to take a deep breath. You should feel no change. You may feel the lower portion of the kidney. Do the same thing on the left side, with the left kidney sitting about one centimeter higher than the right kidney. It should not normally be palpable.

Palpate the aorta, use your thumbs to palpate the aortic pulsation in the upper abdomen. Assess for costovertebral angle tenderness. Place one hand at the costovertebral angle, and the person should feel no pain.

Assess for rebound tenderness to identify peritoneal irritation. To do this hold your hand perpendicular to the abdomen, and push down gently, slowly and deeply, then lift up quickly. If the patient feels rebound tenderness, this is a sign of peritoneal inflammation. Ask where the pain is most intense.

If the patient has a distended abdomen, testing for a fluid wave will help to distinguish between dilated loops of bowel, fat, and free fluid. Have the patient place the ulnar edge of their hand in the umbilical area, mid-line abdomen. You should then place your left hand on the person's right flank, and with your right hand reach across the abdomen and give the left flank a firm shake. If ascites is present, this will generate a fluid wave through the abdomen. A distinct tap on your opposite hand if ascites is present.

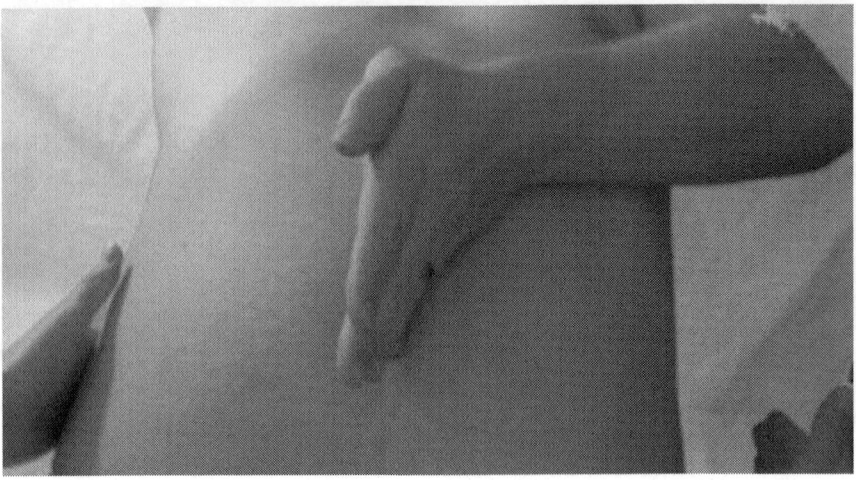

Abnormal Findings

Ascites

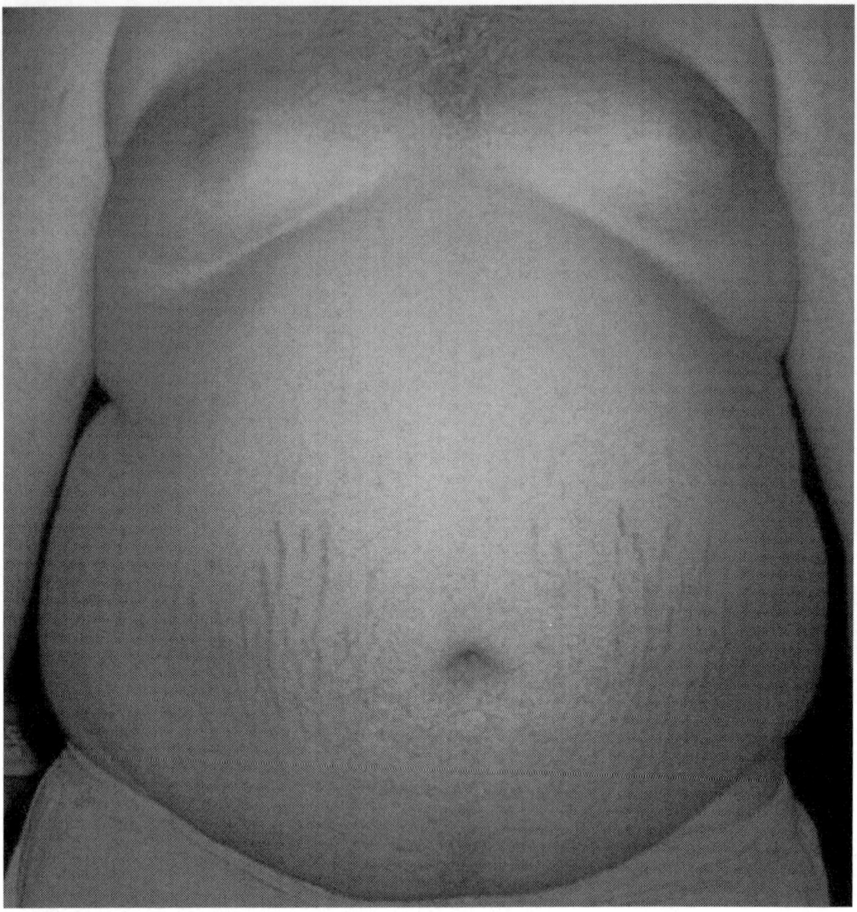

Cullen's Sign

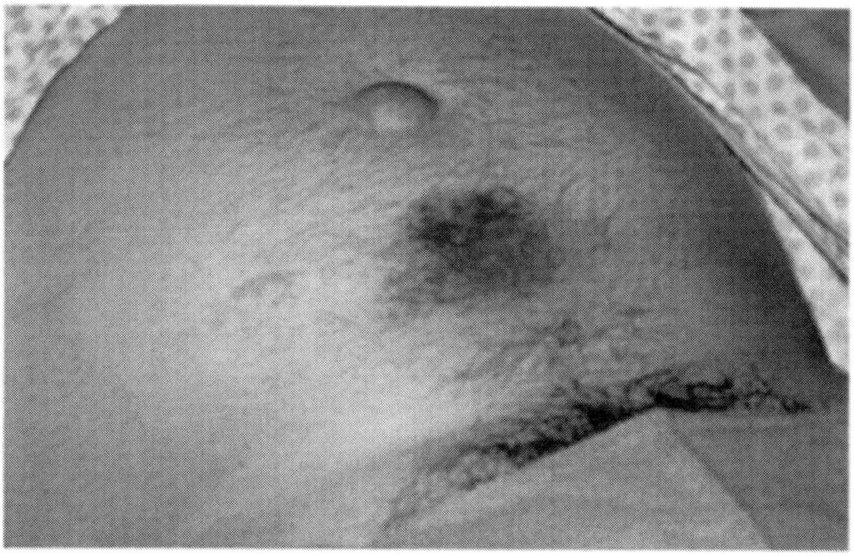

By Herbert L. Fred, MD and Hendrik A. van Dijk (http://cnx.org/content/m14904/latest/) [CC BY 2.0 (http://creativecommons.org/licenses/by/2.0)], via Wikimedia Commons

Musculoskeletal

Anatomy

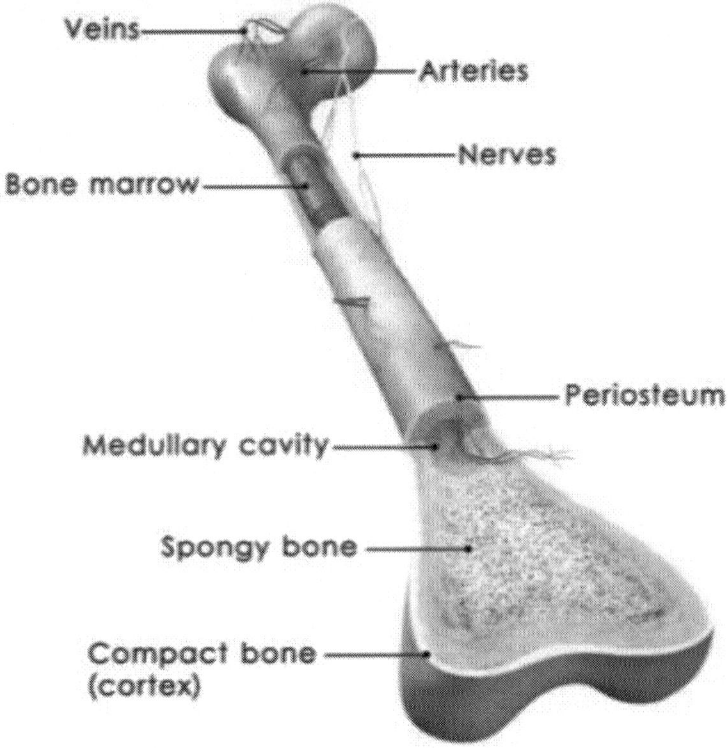

The musculoskeletal system is comprised of bones, joints and muscles. The bones provide support and protection for vital organs in the body. Bones also store minerals like phosphorus and calcium and produce red and white blood cells.

Bones are connected by joints. Synovial joints contain a cavity filled with synovial fluid. Cartilage covers each bone at the joint and ligaments connect the two bones and help strengthen the joint. In certain areas of the body there are fluid filled sacs called bursa that help at points of possible friction: prepatellar bursa of the knee.

Muscles attach to bone via tendons. Muscles are made of actin and myosin filaments that allow for movement via contraction or relaxation of the muscle fibers. There are three different types of muscle: skeletal, smooth, and cardiac.

Skeletal muscle is a voluntary muscle. It is connected to our skeleton via tendons and is involved in movement. Smooth muscle is involuntary and is found within organs of the body. Cardiac muscle is involuntary. It is similar to skeletal muscle, but found in the heart.

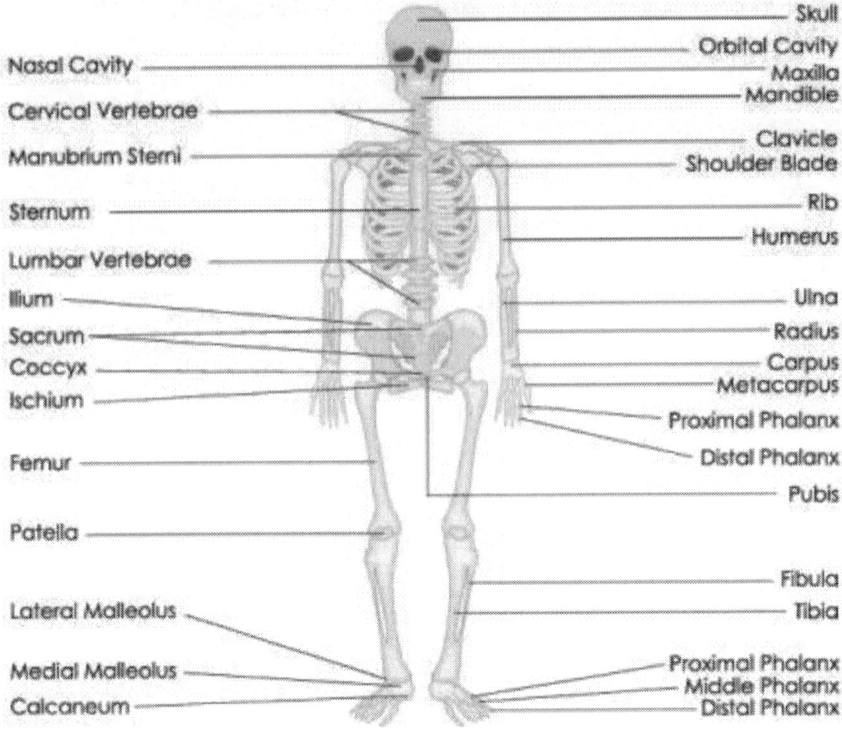

Inspection and Palpation

When assessing the musculoskeletal system, begin with inspection. Inspect corresponding joints, structure, and function of each joint to determine if full range of motion is present. Note the size of each joint, color, swelling, and any masses or deformity on the joint. Palpate the joint and skin to note temperature, as well as musculoskelatal or muscular deformations or swelling at the joints.

Assess range of motion of the joints by asking the patient to do active range of motion in the joint corresponding to the type of joint that it is (flexion, extension, abduction, adduction, pronation, supination, circumduction, elevation, depression, rotation, protraction, retraction, eversion, and inversion). Have the patient attempt these movements in each of their joints.

If the patient is unable to do so, attempt passive range of motion. Assist the patient with passive range of motion. If they are unable to complete passive range of motion exercises, do not force any movements. You can use a goniometer to measure the angles at which the patient is able to move. Joint motion should not cause pain or tenderness, or crepitation.

Assess the cervical spine. Inspect the spine first to see that it is aligned with the head and neck, and that it is centered. Palpate the spine and spinal processes. They should feel firm with no spasms or tenderness.

Ask the patient to touch chin to chest and lift their chin toward the ceiling. Touch each ear toward the corresponding shoulder without lifting the shoulder and turn the chin toward each shoulder. The patient should be able to do these movements equally bilaterally, without any sort of pain.

Assess the upper extremities. Inspect both shoulders, posterior and anteriorly assessing the size, and check for any atrophy, deformity or swelling. Palpate the shoulders and assess that there are no spasms, tenderness, swelling or heat.

To test range of motion in the upper extremities ask patient stand with arms at sides and elbows extended. Have the patient move each arm forward in upward arcs and vertical arcs. They should then rotate the arms internally, behind the back, and place back of hands as high as possible.

Test the strength of the shoulder by asking the person to shrug the shoulders up and place a slight amount of resistance.

Inspect the elbow, inspect the size and contour, notice any sorts of deformity, or swelling, or lesions. Test range of motion by asking the person to bend and straighten the elbow.

Inspect the wrist and hand, noting position, contour and shape. The fingers should lie straight along the same axis as the forearm. There should be no swelling, redness or deformity. The skin should be smooth, the muscle should be full. You should palpate each joint in the wrists and hands.

There should be no bogginess. The surfaces should be smooth. Test range of motion on the wrists and hands by having the patient bend the hand up at the wrist, bend the hand down, and bend the fingers up and down. The patient should be able to have their palms flat, and turn them inward and outward, spread the fingers apart and make a fist, and touch the thumb to each finger on the hand.

Assess the lower extremities. Begin by assessing the hip and the hip joint. Assess that there is symmetry at the level of the iliac crest, and that the patient has a smooth gait.

Lay the patient in a supine position and palpate the hip joints to test for range of motion in the hip. Have the patient raise each leg, with knee extended, bend each knee up to the chest while keeping the other leg straight. The patient should be able to swing the leg laterally then medially with the knee straight. The patient should be able to, in a standing position, swing a straight leg back behind the body.

Next, inspect the knee. Inspect the lower ligament, and inspect the knee shape and contour. There should be no swelling within the knee. Check the quadricep muscle and anterior thigh for any atrophy. Assess range of motion by asking the patient to bend and extend each knee. Have the patient walk. Assesee ambulation as well as range of motion during ambulation.

Assess strength by asking the person to keep the knee flexed while applying a slight amount of pressure.

Inspect the ankle and foot. Compare both feet, the positions of toes and characteristics. Assess for any abnormalities.

Assess the spine. The person should be standing. Place yourself far enough back so that you can see the entire back. Note if the spine is straight by following an imaginary vertical line from head, through the spinous processes and down to the gluteal cleft.

The person's knees should be aligned with the trunk and should be pointing forward. From the side, you should note a normal convex thoracic curve and a concave lumbar curve. You should assess range of motion of the spine by asking the person to bend forward and touch the toes. They should be able to do this in a smooth fashion.

Assess for Homans sign to identify DVT.

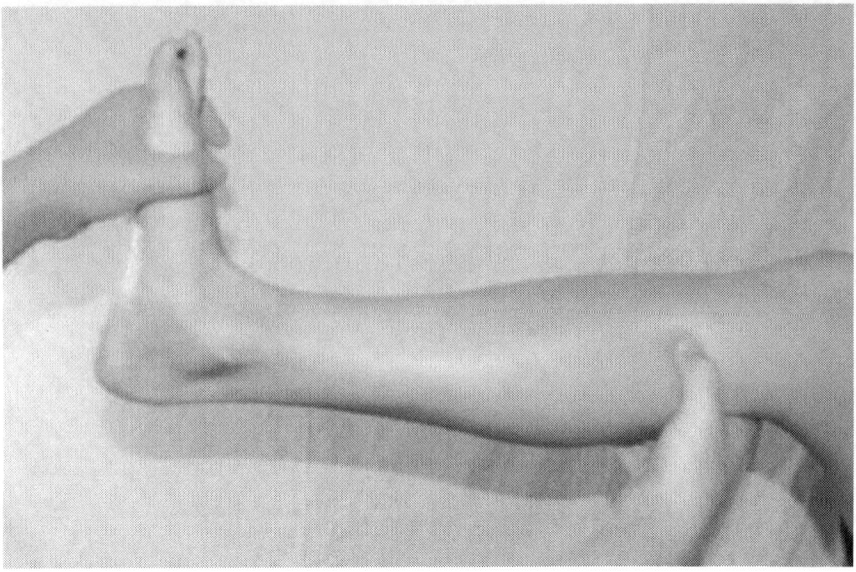

Abnormal Findings

Kyphosis

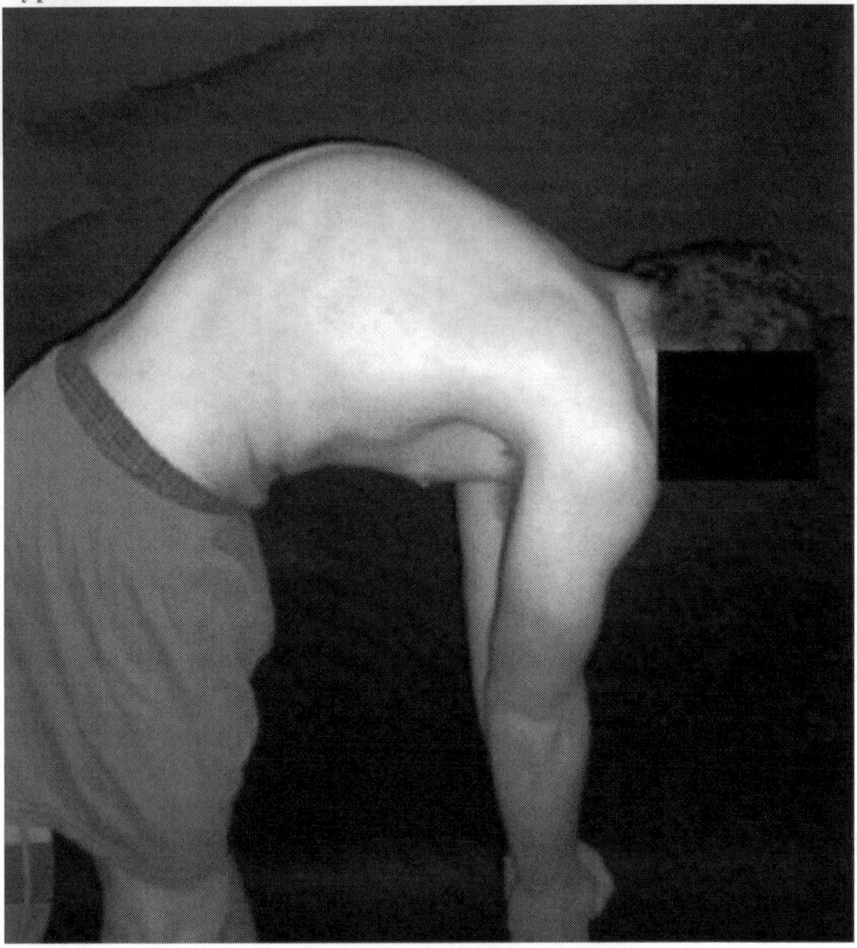

By MusicNewz (Own work this is me) [CC0], via Wikimedia Commons

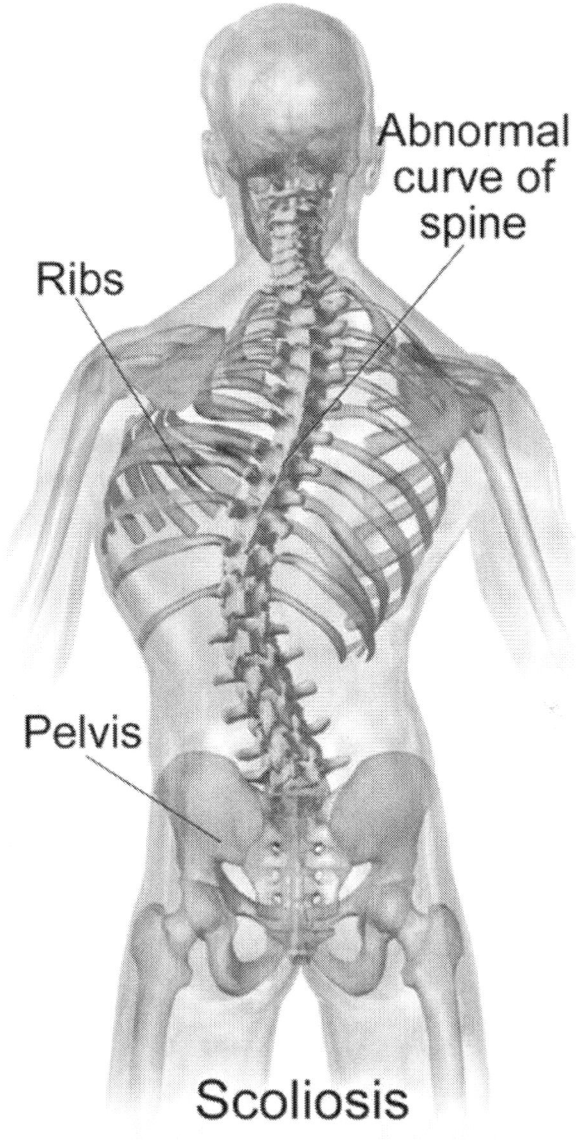

By BruceBlaus. When using this image in external sources it can be cited as: Blausen.com staff. "Blausen gallery 2014". Wikiversity Journal of Medicine.

DOI:10.15347/wjm/2014.010. ISSN 20018762. (Own work) [CC BY 3.0 (http://creativecommons.org/licenses/by/3.0)], via Wikimedia Commons

Kyphosis, Lordosis

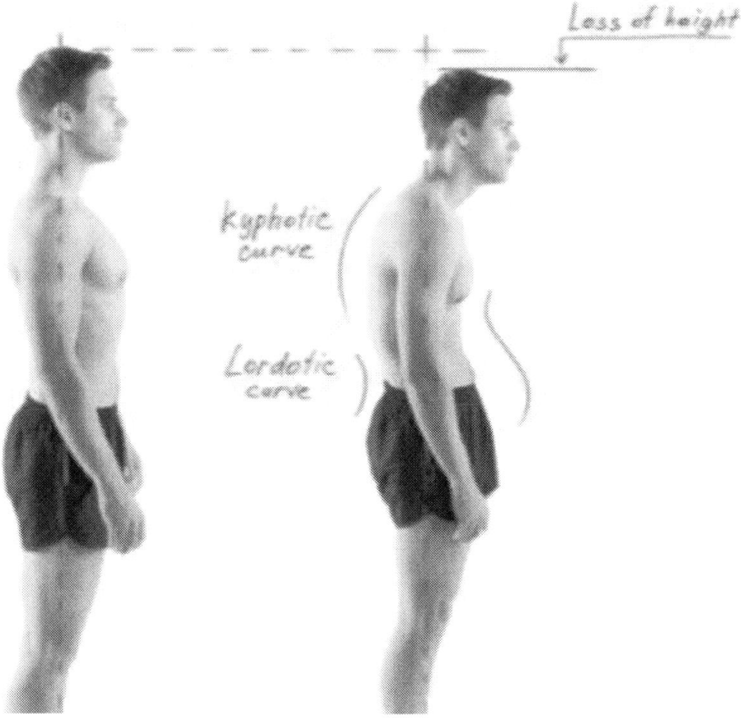

Neurological

Anatomy

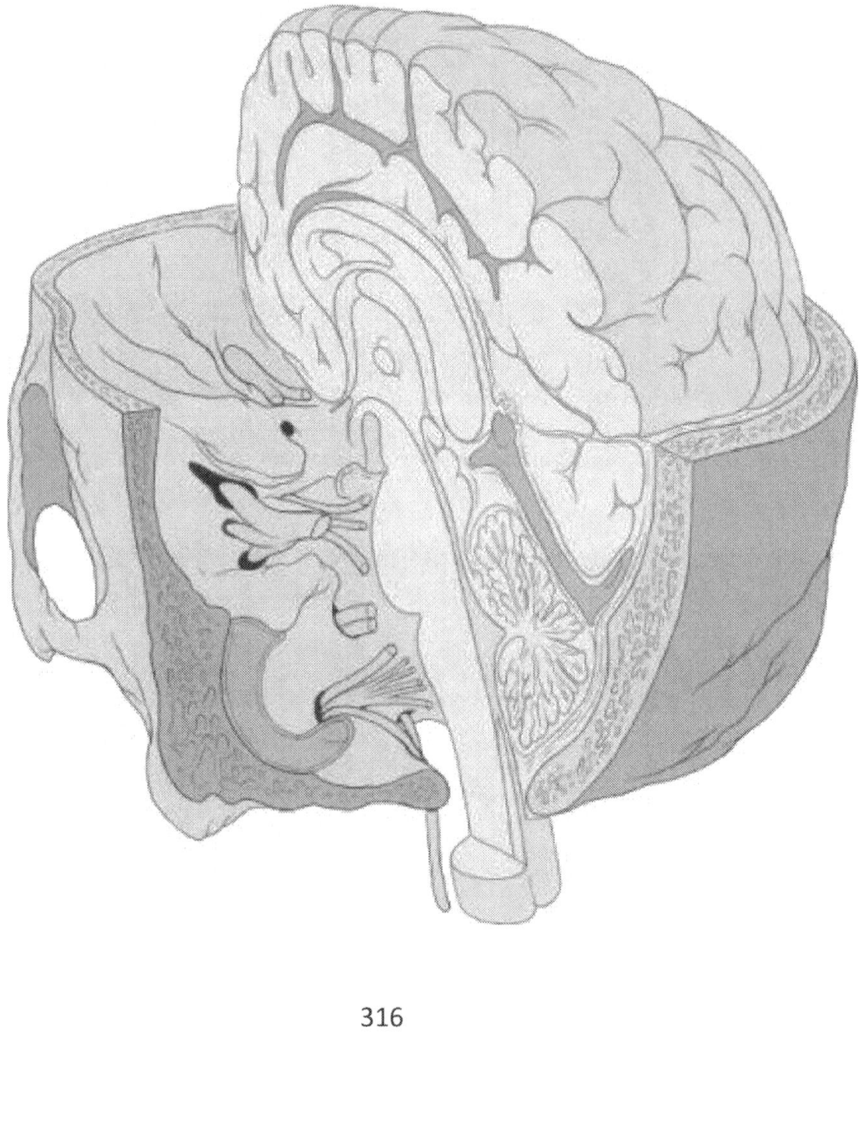

By Patrick J. Lynch, medical illustrator (Patrick J. Lynch, medical illustrator) [CC BY 2.5 (http://creativecommons.org/licenses/by/2.5)], via Wikimedia Commons

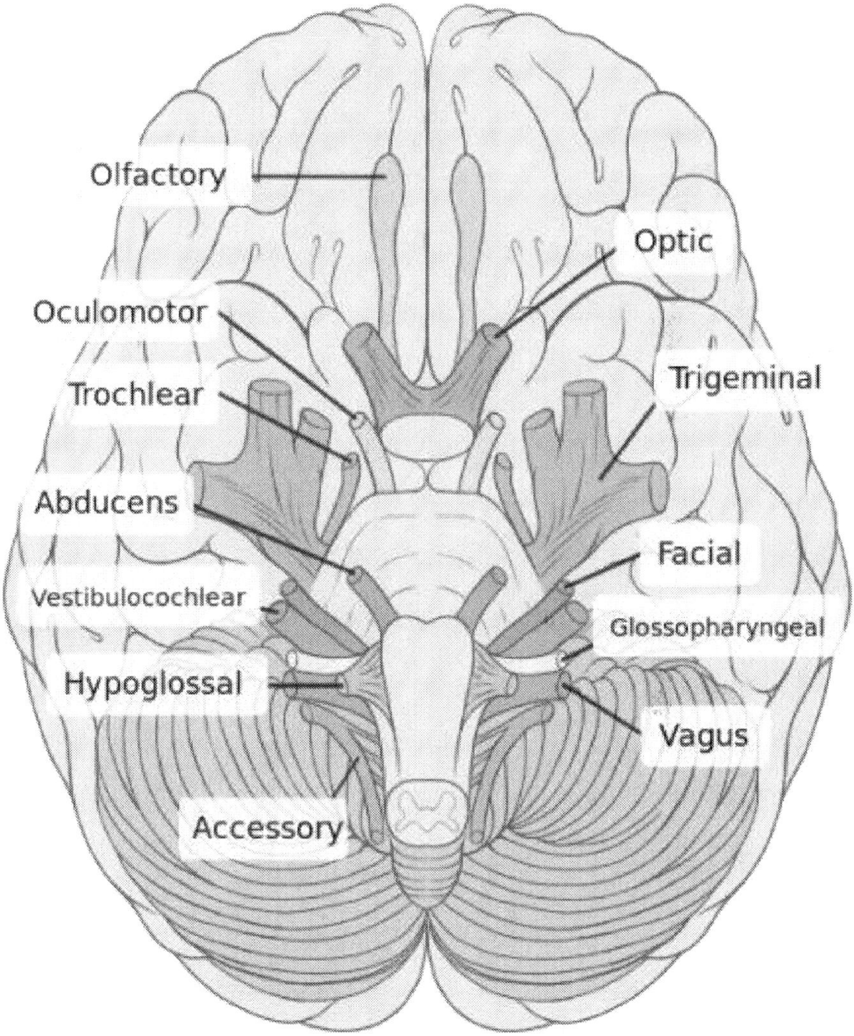

By Brain_human_normal_inferior_view_with_labels_en.svg: *Brain_human_normal_inferior_view.svg: Patrick J. Lynch, medical illustrator derivative

The central nervous system is composed of the brain and spinal column. The brain is encased by the skull and the spinal column by the vertebrae. The primary cell of the CNS is the neuron which has unique capabilities. The brain consists of a right and left hemisphere connected by a group of nerves called the corpus callosum. Each hemisphere contains a frontal lobe, temporal lobe, parietal lobe, and occipital lobe.

In the middle of the brain is the thalamus. It relays sensory signals to the cerebral cortex. It is also involved in sleep wake cycles.

The hypothalamus located just below the thalamus plays a role in hunger, thirst, sleep, emotions, temperature, and stimulation of the pituitary.

Posterior to the hypothalamus is the midbrain and below that is the pons. They are involved in motor and sensory functions.

The cerebellum is associated with balance and equilibrium, coordination, muscle tone. The medulla helps regulate respiratory, gastrointestinal and heart functions.

There are 12 pairs of cranial nerves and 31 pairs of spinal nerves. The cranial nerves originate in the brain while the spinal nerves originate from different sections of the spinal cord. The spinal nerves are further classified based on location: sacral spinal nerves, thoracic spinal nerves etc.

Neurons are the primary cell found in the central nervous system. They have a unique shape that allows them to be quick and efficient communicators. This allows us to instantly sense pain in our hand from a hot stove.

Neurons are capable of transmitting electric impulse as well as communicating chemically via neurotransmitters.

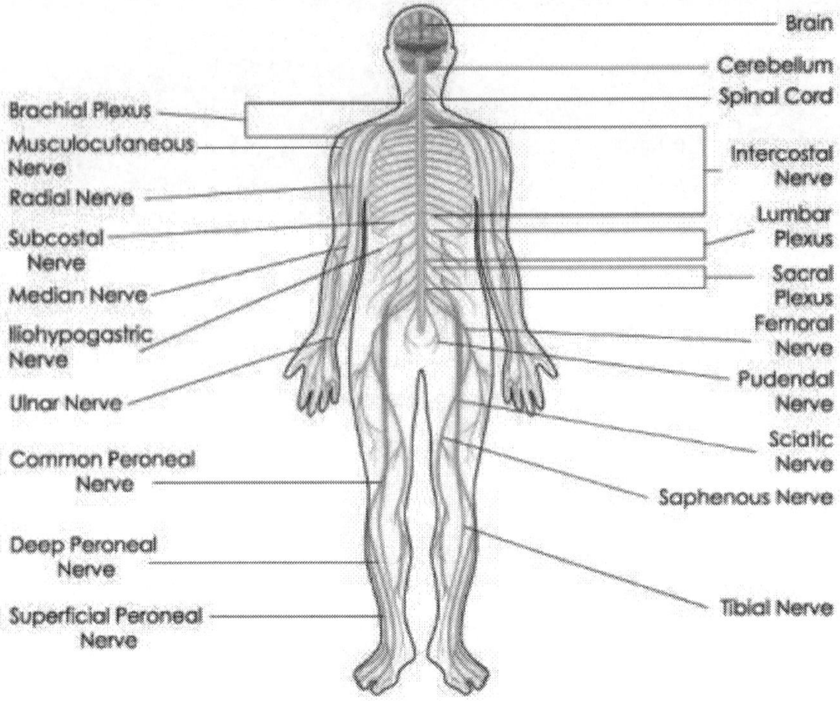

Level of Consciousness

When conducting the neurological system assessment, begin by assessing level of consciousness. Is the person alert, awake, and aware of the stimulus in their environment? Are they oriented to person, time, situation and place? What's their facial expression? What is the quality of their speech? What is their general mood and affect?

Assess the appearance of the patient, position, posture as well as dress and grooming.

Assess cognitive function. Is the person oriented to time, place and person? Assess attention span. Are they able to focus on the interview? Are they able to focus on you and what is being done at the moment? What is their recent memory? Are they able to recall why they're in the hospital, what happened, and what brought them to the hospital?

Assess remote memory, past events, birth dates? What is their judgment? Assess thought processes. Is the person making sense? Are they able to make sense of what is happening? Assess their perceptions, ask them questions about their perception of the world.

Screen them for suicidal thoughts. Ask if they have any thoughts of hurting themselves.

Further assess neurological status. Are they alert? Meaning, are they awake and readily aroused? Are they fully aware of what's happening? Are they lethargic or somnolent, not fully alert, drift into sleep, requiring stimulation? Are they obtunded, sleeping most of the time, very difficult to arouse? Are they in a stupor, responding only to vigorous shaking?

Are they in a coma, completely unconscious? Each institution might have different definitions and states for level of consciousness, so it is important to understand how your hospital and your organization determines level of consciousness.

Test cranial nerves. Test cranial nerve II the optic nerve by testing visual acuity. Assess cranial nerves II, IV, and VI, ocular motor, trochlear and abducens nerves. Assess pupil size, the regularity, equality, reaction to light. Are they equal round and reactive to light? This is known as PERRLA (**P**upils **E**qual **R**ound **R**eactive to **L**ight). Assess for extra ocular movements by assessing for the six cardinal positions.

Assess cranial nerve V, the trigeminal nerve, by assessing motor function. Palpate the temporal masseter muscles as the person clenches their teeth. With the person's eyes closed, test light touch sensation by touching the forehead, cheeks and chin, and having the person state when they feel that they're being touched.

Test the facial nerve, cranial nerve VII, by motor function. Note facial symmetry as the person responds, as they smile, frown, close eyes tightly, and lift eyebrows, to show teeth. Assess for symmetry on each side.

Olfactory-**S**ensory

Optic-**S**ensory

Oculomotor-**M**otor

Trochlear-**M**otor

Trigeminal-**B**oth

Abducens-**M**otor

Facial-**B**oth

Vestibulocochlear-**S**ensory

Glossopharyngeal-**B**oth

Vagus-**B**oth

Accessory-**M**otor

Hypoglossal-**M**otor

Inspect and palpate the motor system. Assess cerebellar function by assessing gait and balance. Is the person able to walk in a smooth gait, is it rhythmic, effortless, and coordinated? Use the Romberg test by asking the person to stand up with their feet together. Have the person stand with their feet together and close their eyes, are they able to stand in a completely balanced and coordinated fashion for 20 seconds.

Assess the sensory system. The person needs to be alert, comfortable and cooperative in order to do this. Assess for superficial pain by using something sharp and something dull to touch the patient, determine if the patient is able to distinguish between sharp and dull.

Assess stereognosis by placing different objects in the patient's hand with their eyes closed, and determine if they can distinguish between items like paperclips, keys, and coins.

Assess reflexes. Reflexes are graded from zero to four: zero, no response, to four plus, very brisk, hyperactive.

- 0: no response
- 1+: diminished
- 2+: average or normal

- 3+: brisker than average
- 4+: very brisk, hyperactive, clonus, indicative of disease.

Assess the bicep reflex, which will test C5 and C6.

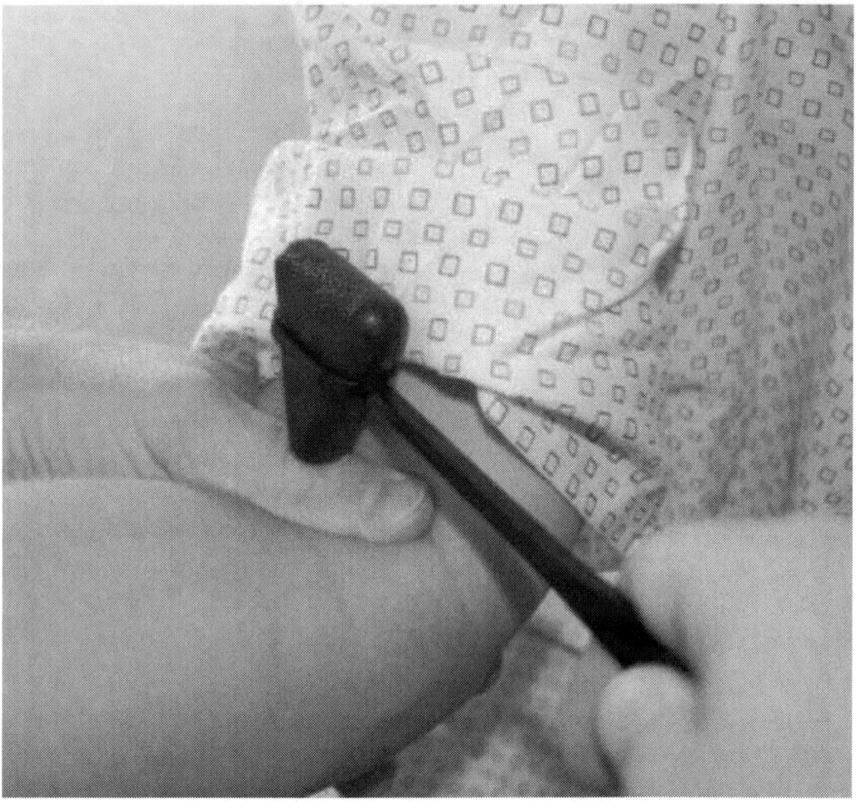

Assess the tricep reflex, which would be C7 and C8.

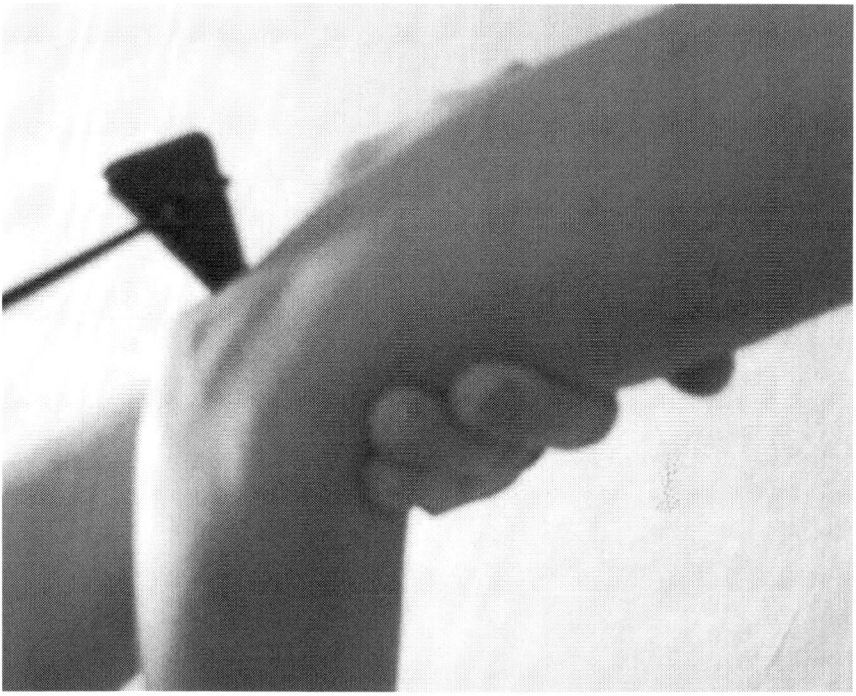

Assess patellar reflex, L2 to L4. The achilles reflex tests L5 to S2.

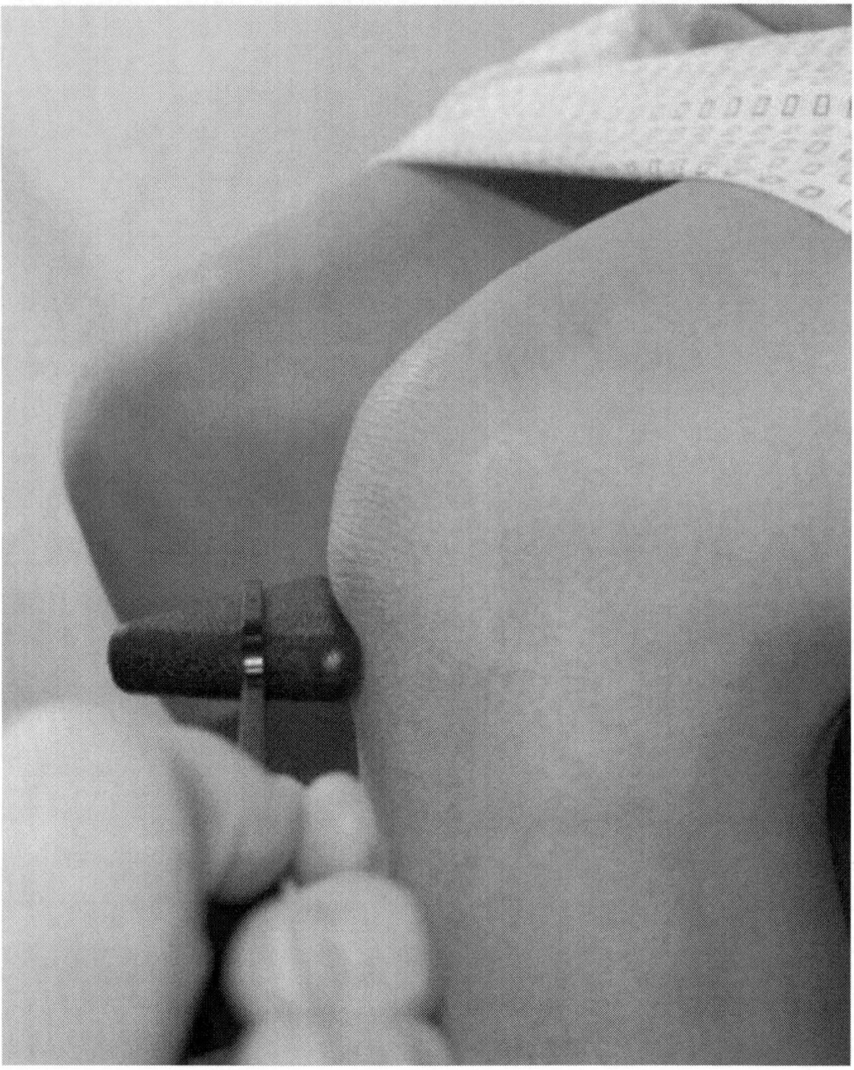

Assess achilles reflex.

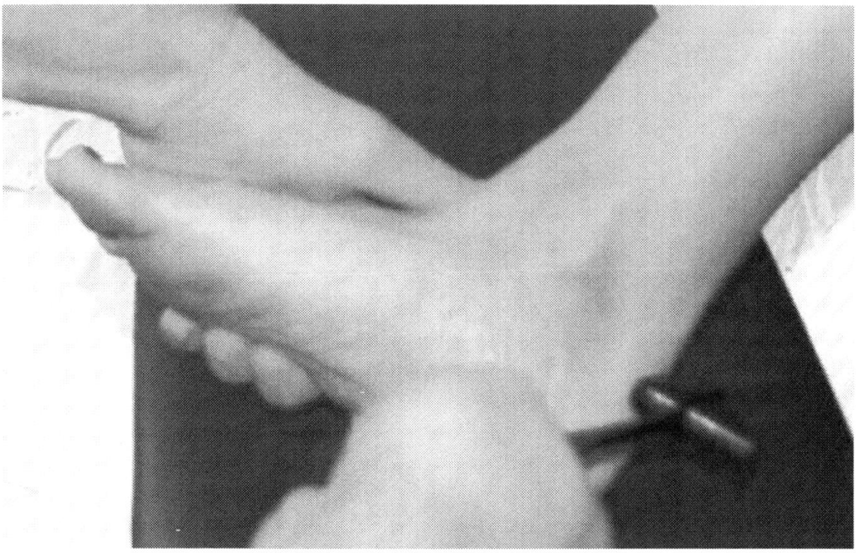

Assess for Babinski reflex by drawing a light stroke from the person's heel to the person's toes in the shape of a J. The normal response is the plantar flexion of the toes, which would be bringing the toes forward toward the stimulus. A positive Babinski reflex would indicate upper motor neuron disease.

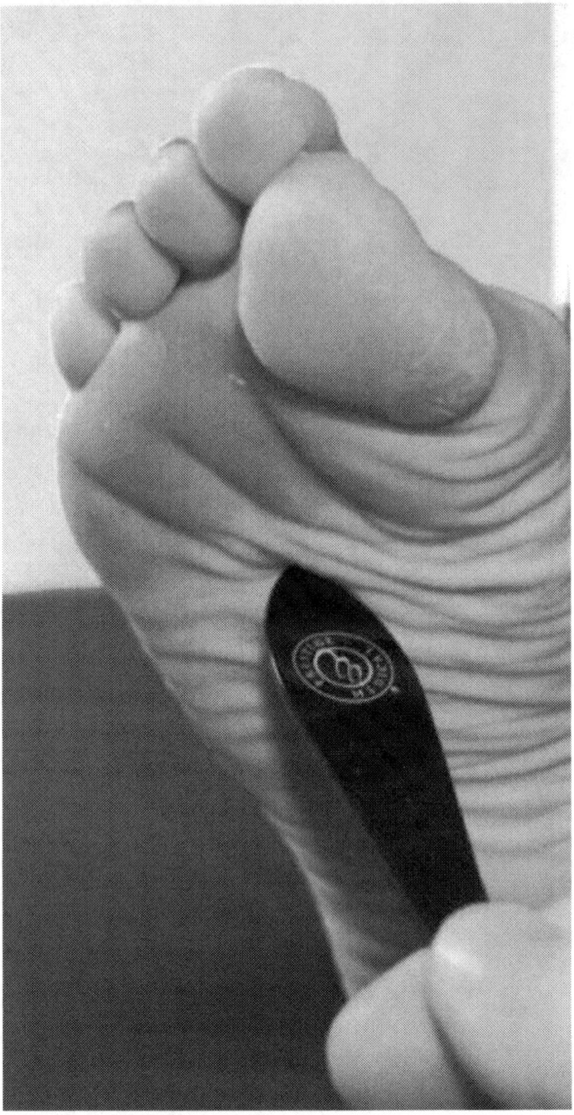

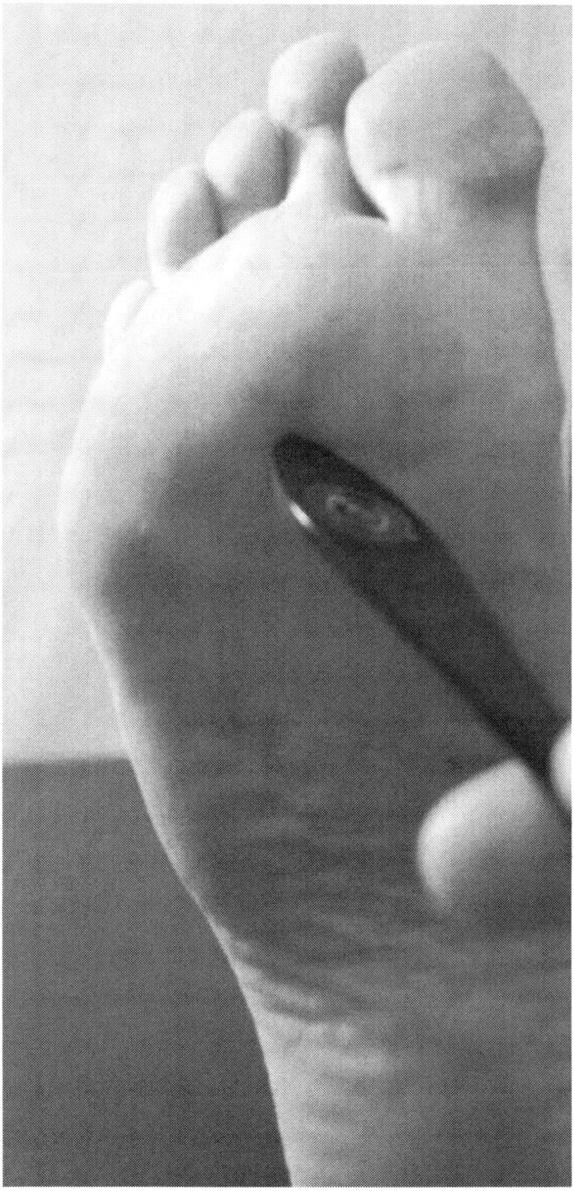

Abnormal Findings

Bells Palsy

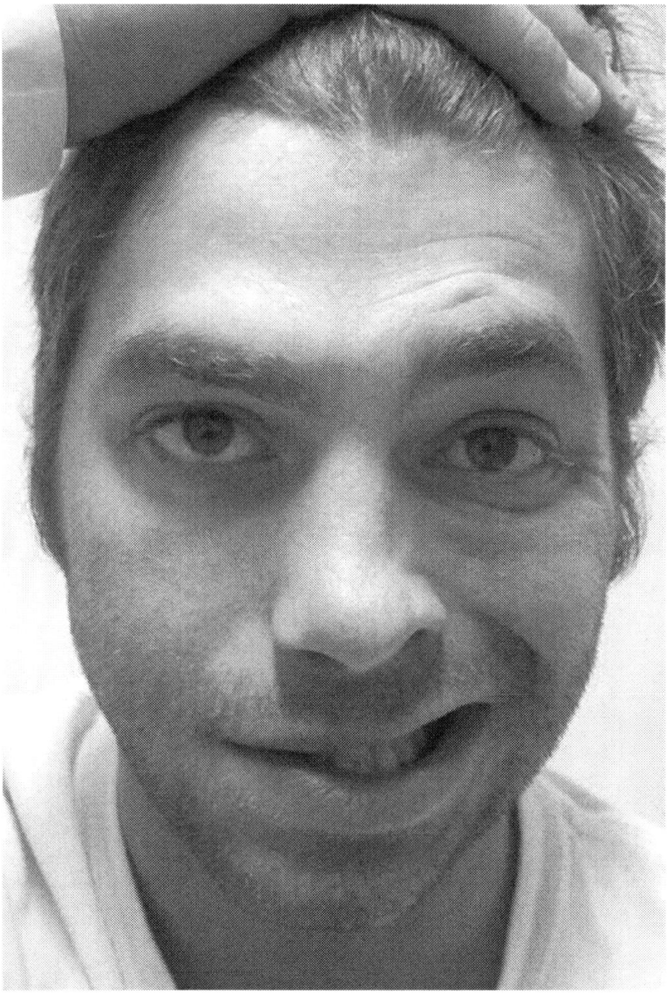

By James Heilman, MD (Own work) [CC BY-SA 3.0 (http://creativecommons.org/licenses/by-sa/3.0) or GFDL (http://www.gnu.org/copyleft/fdl.html)], via Wikimedia Commons

Dystonia

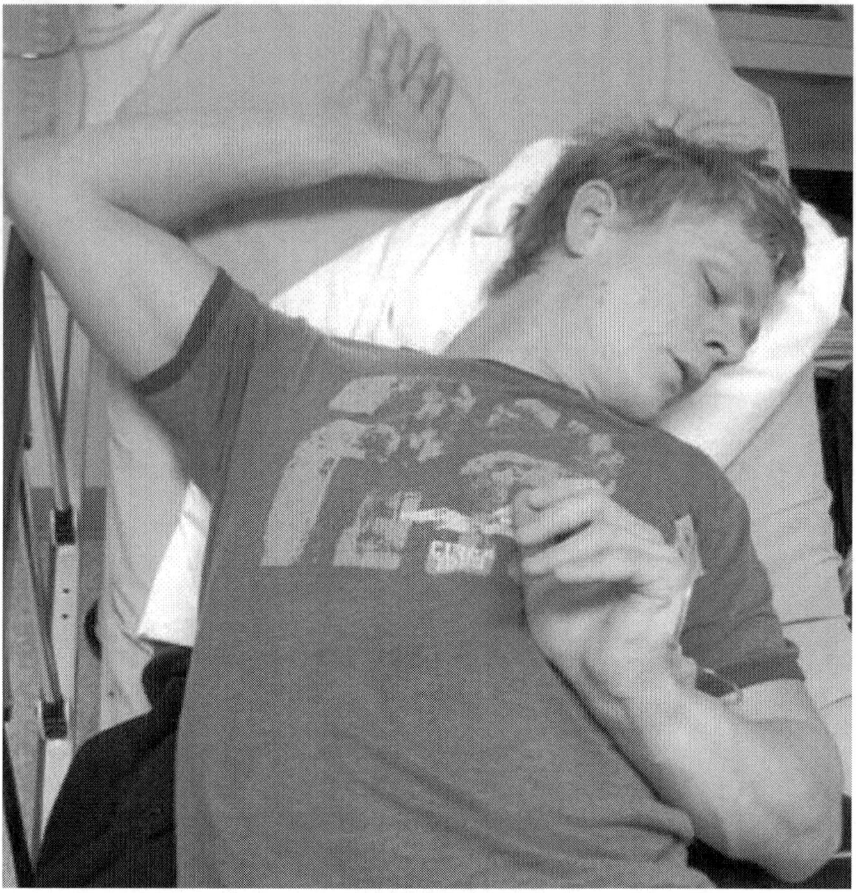

By James Heilman, MD (Own work) [CC BY-SA 3.0 (http://creativecommons.org/licenses/by-sa/3.0) or GFDL (http://www.gnu.org/copyleft/fdl.html)], via Wikimedia Commons

Meningitis (neck stiffness)

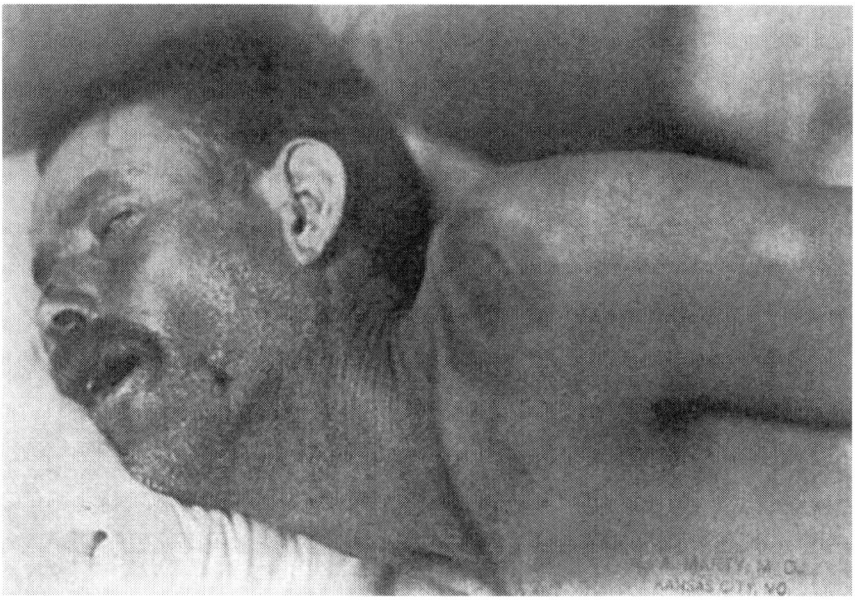

Positive Babinski Sign

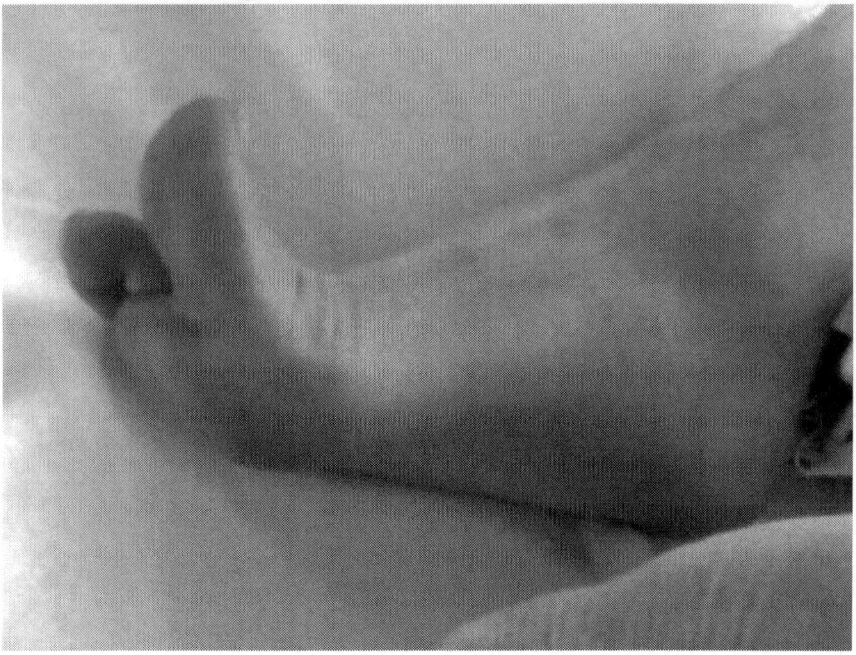

Male Genitourinary

Anatomy

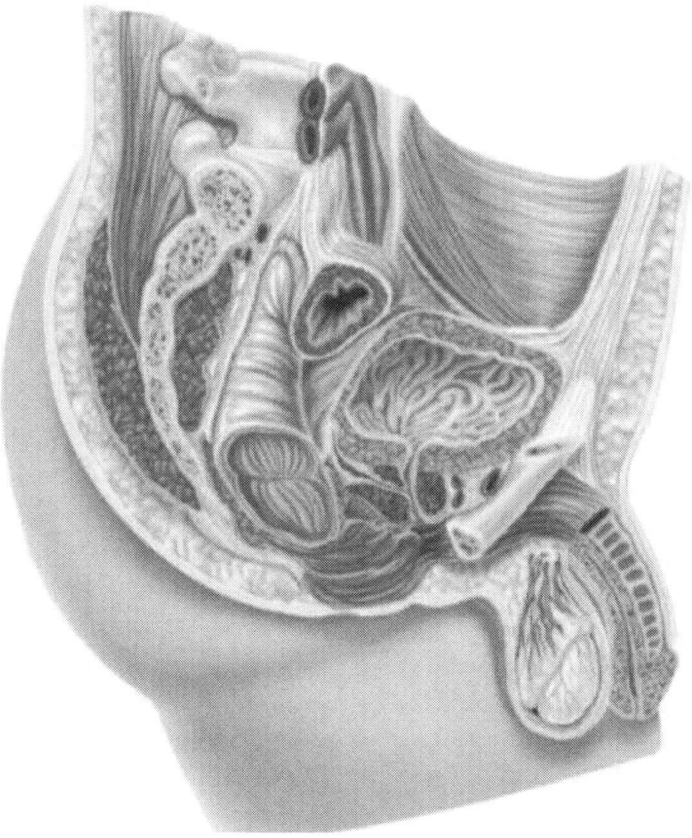

The male reproductive system consists of the scrotum, penis, testis, epidydimis, and vas deferens. The urethra runs through the center of the penis and ends at the tip where waste is removed. The scrotum is a loose sac behind the penis that holds the testis.

Above the testis lie the epididymis which stores sperm that is produced in the testes. The epididymis combines with the vas deferens. The vas deferens with several other vessels is called the spermatic cord.

Puberty typically begins between 9 1/2 and 13 1/3 years of age.

The prostrate is found in males, located just below the bladder. It secretes and alkaline fluid that helps maintain sperm viability. It is divided into two lobes by a groove called the median sulcus. Two glands called seminal vesicles secrete a fluid that has fructose to feed the sperm.

Inspection and Palpation

Inspect and palpate the scrotum. Scrotal size will vary depending on patient and room temperature. Asymmetry is normal with the left scrotal half lower than the right. There should be no lesions or cysts.

Palpate each half between your thumb and first two fingers. Testis should feel oval. They should be freely movable and slightly tender. There should be no other scrotal content

Inspect and palpate for hernia by inspecting the inguinal region for bulge. Palpate the inguinal canal while the patient strains down. Inspect here for inguinal lymph nodes by palpating along the vertical chain within the upper inner thigh.

Instruct the patient to conduct a testicular self-examination once a month, the best time for this being after a warm shower.

Prostate Examination

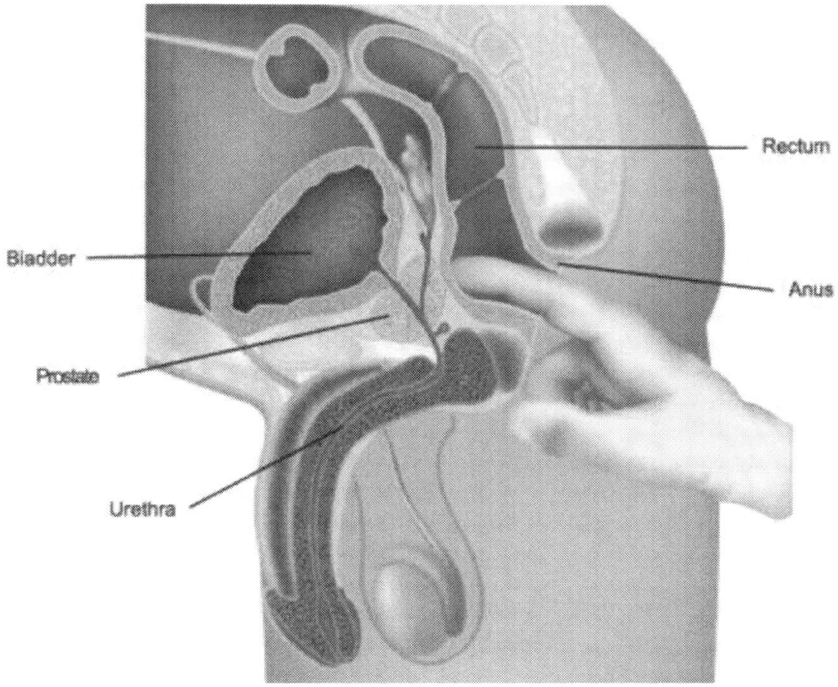

Palpate the prostate gland by pressing into the gland to note the size. The size should be about two-and-a-half centimeters long, about four centimeters wide and should not protrude more than one centimeter into the rectum. Its shape should be heart shape and the surface should be smooth. It should be elastic, and rubbery, and slightly movable. There should be no tenderness on palpation. As the examination finger is withdrawn assess any signs of bright blood or mucous on the glove. At this time test stool for occult blood.

Female Genitourinary

Anatomy

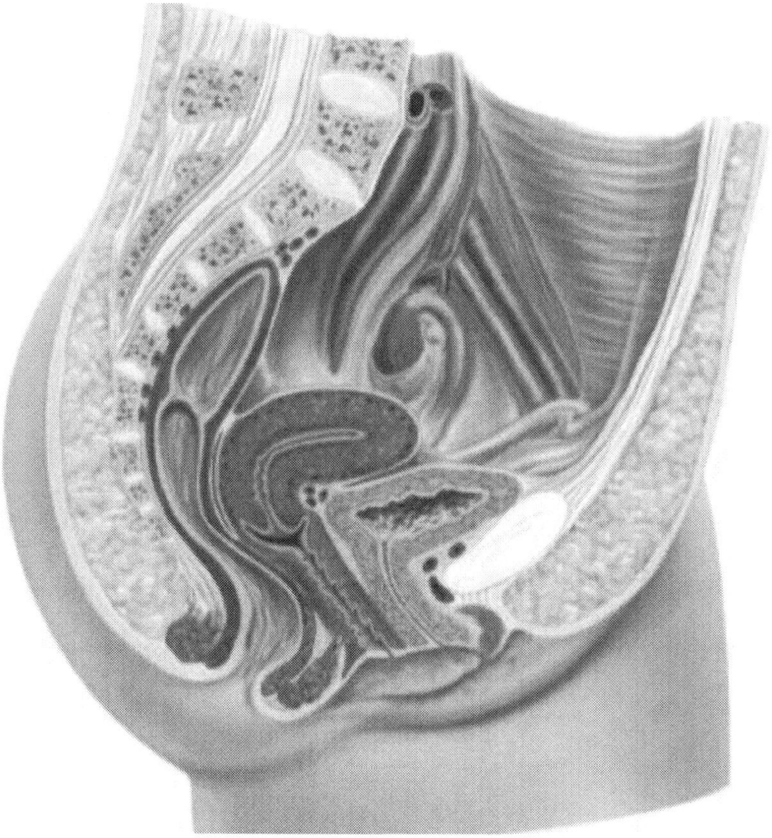

The female reproductive system includes the breasts, vulva, mons pubis, vestibule, clitoris, vagina, cervix, uterus, ovaries and fallopian tubes.

The mons pubis is a pad of adipose tissue and covers the symphisis pubis. The vestibule is surrounded by the labia minora and labia majora. It includes the urethral meatus and vaginal opening.

The clitoris is located anterior to the urethral meatus which is anterior to the vaginal opening. Two bartholin's glands sit next to the vaginal opening and secret mucus during intercourse. The vagina extends up into the pelvis and ends at the uterine cervix.

Two fallopian tubes extend from the top of the uterus up near the ovaries. Ovaries develop ova or eggs and produce hormones.

Puberty in girls starts between 8 1/2 and 13 years of age. Signs include breast and pubic hair growth, menarche.

The primary function of the female breast is milk production after childbirth. The breast lie above the pectoralis muscle between rib 2 and 6.

The axillary Tail of Spence is where a small section of breast tissue extends up into the axilla. The breast is made predominantly of adipose tissue, with some grandular tissue and 4 lactiferous ducts that lead toward the nipple.

The breast tissue is held in place by Cooper's ligaments that connect to chest muscle. The breast is divided into 4 sections: upper outer, lower outer, upper inner, lower inner. The central axillary nodes, pectoral nodes, subscapular nodes, and lateral nodes of the lymphatic system all provide drainage from the breast.

Inspection and Palpation

When conducting the assessment of the female genital urinary system, you should note skin color, hair distribution.

The labia majora should be symmetrical and well-formed. There should be no lesions or cysts. With a gloved hands, separate the labia majora to inspect the clitoris. The labia minora should be dark pink,moist and symmetric. The perineum should be smooth while the anus has coarse skin with increase pigmentation.

Palpate the clitoral gland. Assess the urethra and Skenes gland. Insert your finger into the vagina and apply pressure up and out. There should be no pain upon doing this.

Assess the Bartholin's gland by palpating the posterior part of the labia majora.

Inspect the genitalia by using a speculum for examination. With the speculum inserted, inspect the cervix. The color should be pink and even within a female who is not pregnant. The position should be midline. The size is about two-and-a-half centimeters. The os is small and round in women who have never been pregnant, in parous woman it is a horizontal, irregular slit. It should be smooth.

If there are secretions depending on menstrual cycle, they should be odorless.

Obtain cervical cultures (Pap smear or Papanicolaou smear) to screen for cervical cancer.

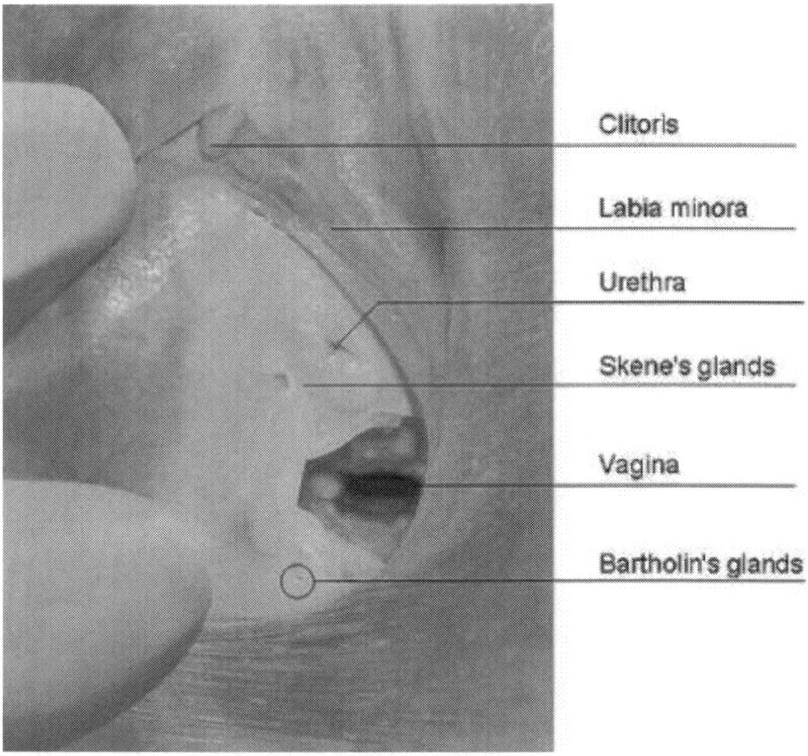

Bimanual Examination

With the woman in a lithotomy position, one hand will be placed on the abdomen. With the other hand insert two fingers into the vagina. Palpate the vaginal wall. It should be smooth with no areas of induration or tenderness. It should feel consistent throughout and be evenly rounded, with the cervix able to move from side-to-side.

With the abdominal hand push the pelvic organs closer to your intervaginal fingers to palpate. Palpate the uterine wall. It normally feels firm and smooth. The uterus should be moved freely and non tender.

Conduct a recto-vaginal examination to assess the recto-vaginal septum, posterior uterine wall, cul-de-sac, and rectum. This may feel uncomfortable to the woman and feel as though she were having a bowel movement. With one hand, insert one finger into the anus and one into the vagina, and with the other hand to apply pressure to the abdomen.

The recto-vaginal septum should feel smooth and thin. The uterine wall and fundus should feel firm and smooth. As rectal finger is withdrawn assess for any signs of blood.

Breasts and Axilla

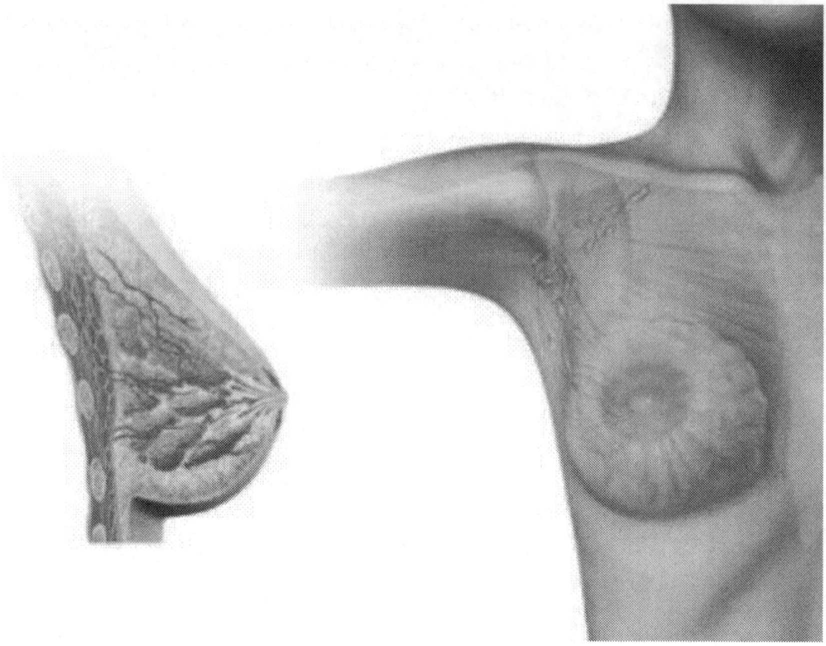

Inspection and Palpation

Inspect the breast. Note asymmetry and size. There may be a slight amount of asymmetry in the size of the breast which is normal. The skin should be smooth. There should be no lesions, or dimpling, or redness. There should be no edema.

There should be no bulging, discoloration or edema in lymphatic draining areas. The nipples should be symmetrically located and should usually protrude although some may be flat or inverted. If an inverted nipple is noted, question the patient if that is new occurrence or preexisting.

Assess for retraction by asking the woman to lift both arms above her head, both breasts should move up symmetrically. Ask the patient to place her hands on her hips and push her two palms together. There will be slight lifting of both breasts.

Inspect and palpate the axilla. Inspect the skin for any rash or infection. Lift the patients arm and support it yourself so that her muscles relax. Reach your fingers into the axilla and move them firmly down in each direction. The lymph nodes are generally not palpable and there should be no tenderness when you palpate.

Palpate the breast. Ask the patient to lay in a supine position with a small pad under the side to be palpated. Use the pads of your first three fingers and make a gentle rotation movement on the breast. Palpate from the nipple and move outward, feeling for any nodules. Make note of any discharge.

Note the location, size, shape, consistency, skin color and tenderness of any lumps or masses.

Instruct the patient to conduct a breast self-examination or BSE. The best time for this is right after the menstrual period or the fourth through seventh day of the menstrual cycle.

When assessing the male breast, inspect it and note any lumps or swelling. Gynecomastia is enlargement of the breast tissue. There should be no nodules or swelling in the male breast.

Lymphatic System

Anatomy

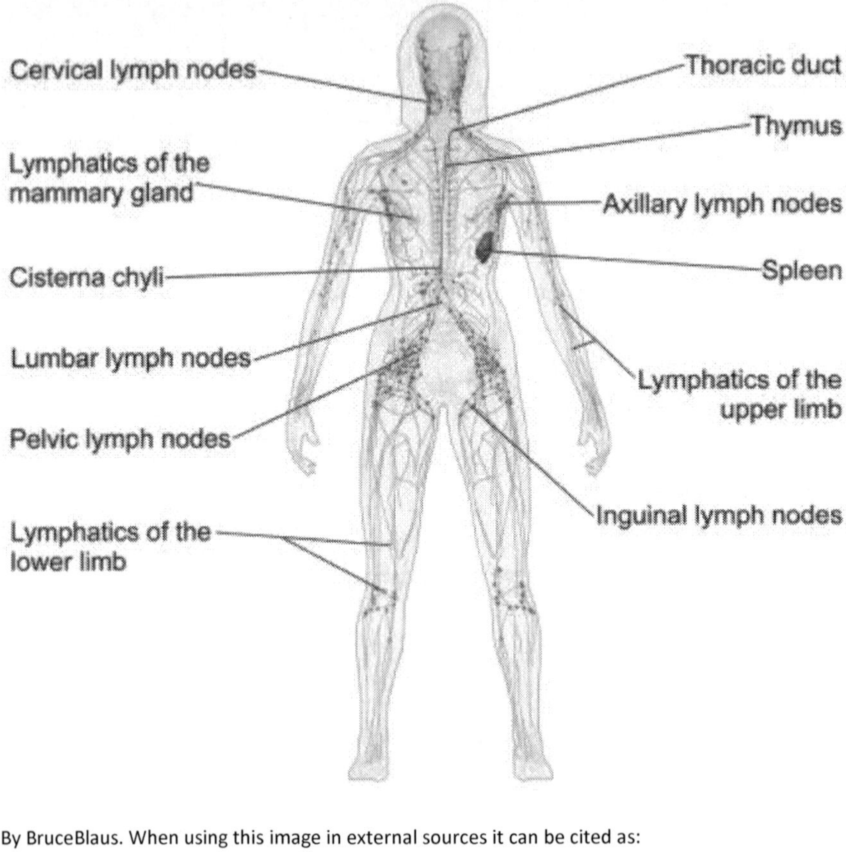

By BruceBlaus. When using this image in external sources it can be cited as: Blausen.com staff. "Blausen gallery 2014". Wikiversity Journal of Medicine. DOI:10.15347/wjm/2014.010. ISSN 20018762. (Own work) [CC BY 3.0 (http://creativecommons.org/licenses/by/3.0)], via Wikimedia Commons

The lymphatic system is a transport system like the peripheral vascular system, however the vessels are separate. The lymph system is composed of lymph vessels, lymph nodes, lymph ducts, and lymph nodules.

When blood is transported throughout the body, plasma from the blood flows into interstitial spaces. To prevent excess build up, the lymph system is there to drain excess fluid and plasma protein.

Lymph is collected in vessels and drains into different lymph nodes in the body where it is filtered and microbes killed. Lymph is then sent to lymph ducts which deposit it into veins to become part of the plasma in the blood supply.

Lymph is very similar to plasma in the blood. The head and neck drain into the cervical lymph nodes. The breast and upper arm are drained by the axillary lymph nodes. The hand and lower arm drain into the epitrochlear lymph node, and the lower extremity drains into the inguinal nodes. Lymph nodules like the thymus and spleen do not connect directly with rest of the lymph system and help protect the body from external pathogens.

Appendix (Resources)

Head to Toe Assessment Video Series

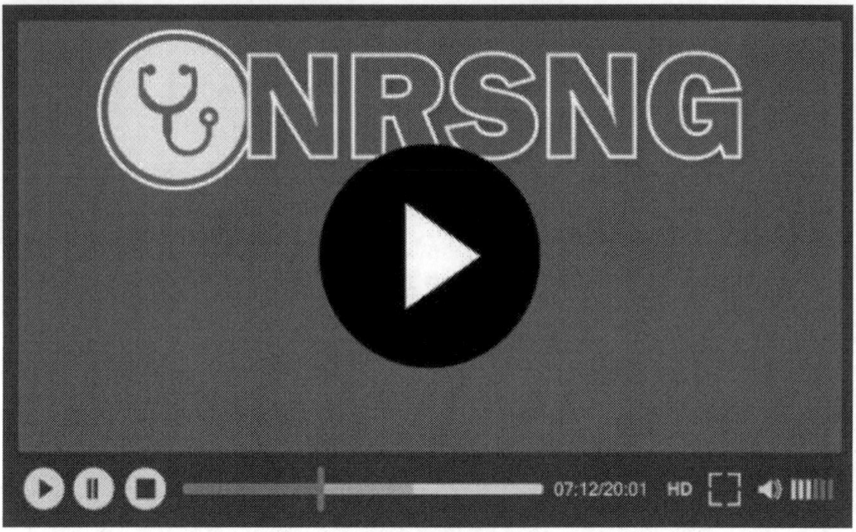

Visit: YouTube.com/user/nrsngcom for a 6 part Physical Assessment Video Series

Clinical Assistant (Assessment Tool and Organizer)

Use this 2 page PDF tool to complete your head to toe assessment and to better organize your clinical day. Visit **gum.co/IaoG** to download for free. If you would like to donate a buck or two that would be appreciated otherwise just type "0" in the amount box.

Clinical Assistant

Created by: Jon Haws NRSNG.com

Reason for hospitalization:

Focused Assessment:

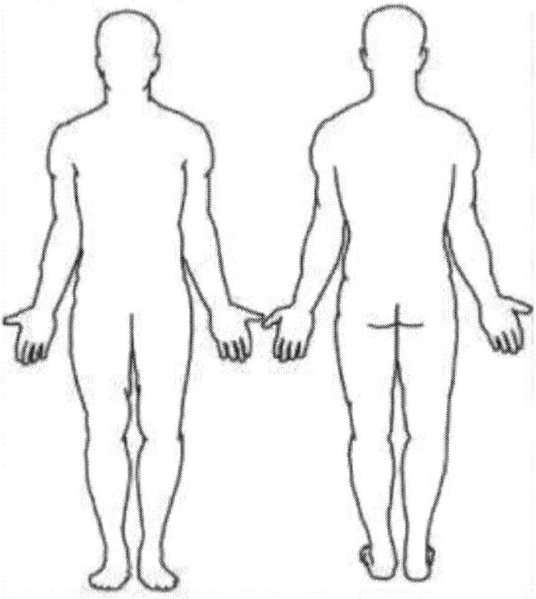

Assessment Notes:

Consultations/Tests:

Patient Medications:			
Name	Reason	Considerations	Time

H&P (History and Physical) Examples

These example H&P documents from the University of North Carolina Medical School provide an excellent resource in learning how to extract the MOST important information and how to write a nursing report. They were a wonderful resource while I was in nursing school.

http://goo.gl/tjvEWb

Handoff Report and Assessment Sheet

One of the key components of a complete assessment is a good report. I have found that new nurses have a hard time organizing their handoff report. This is always one area that I focus on with new nurses.

To help them organize their thoughts I have created the attached 2 page PDF worksheet. By simply working through this sheet you will not only be able to provide a better handoff report, but you will also organize the thoughts in your own head . . . leading to more focused patient care.

NRSNG
where nurses learn

Handoff Report and Assessment Sheet

Name	Age	Allergies	Code	DX	Background	PMH	PSH
Doctors:							

Neurological

Orientation	
Pupils	
Extremities	
Follows Commands	
Speech Clarity	
Behavior	
Sensation	
NIH	

Repiratory

O2 Delivery	
Normal Sats	
Lung Sounds	

Cardiac

Rhythm, rate, trends	
BP trends	
Medication available for control	
Pulse location, strength, cap refill	
Edema	
SCDs, TEDS, VTE Prophylaxis	
Fluids/Drips	
Temps	

Visit: https://gumroad.com/l/pTOxE

References

Jarvis, C. (2008). *Physical examination & health assessment* (5th ed.). St. Louis, Mo.: Saunders/Elsevier.

Porth, C. (2005). *Pathophysiology: Concepts of altered health states* (7th ed.). Philadelphia: Lippincott Williams & Wilkins.

LAB VALUES

63 Must Know Labs for Nurses

Introduction

Providing comprehensive care for patients requires that all clinicians are competent in the interpretation of laboratory data.

Being able to identify abnormal signs and symptoms in patients, including abnormal diagnostic and laboratory data is required of nurses desiring to provide truly holistic care for their patients.

While the duty of diagnosing and ordering procedures based on data lies on the physician, nurses should verse themselves in lab values, their meanings, normal ranges, and the purpose for each test being ordered.

By understanding lab data and taking the time to assess patient's lab values it becomes possible to participate as part of the interdisciplinary team to affect patient outcomes.

This book is not intended to be used as a means of diagnosing or treating patients and should not take the place of thorough clinical assessment, sound judgment, and institutional guidelines. Normal laboratory data may vary slightly from institution to institution. This book is simply a guide in understanding commonly ordered laboratory data.

This is by no means a comprehensive guide of all available lab tests. There are literally countless clinical tests available to diagnose and treat various conditions. This guide covers some of the most common tests that will be ordered on patients and those tests that should be understood in preparation for passing the boards.

Educating patients on the purpose of tests and the results will lead to greater patient satisfaction and, more importantly will make your patients active participates in their health. Simple education on the purpose for tests and normal ranges can help ease patients' anxiety and aid them in gaining confidence with the entire medical team.

Standard Precautions

As with all procedures conducted within the health care setting, it is essential that nurses maintain standard precautions in all patient contact. Transmission of disease from patient to nurse or between patients can be kept to a minimum through basic adherence to standard precautions. The CDC outlines the basics behind standard precautions on their website which can be viewed here: http://goo.gl/pVAhtZ.

Key Components of Standard Precautions:

- Hand Hygiene
- Proper Use of PPE
- Injection Safety
- Environmental Cleaning
- Medical Equipment
- Respiratory Hygiene

Areas where nurses tend to break standard precautions with patients include the following:

- Not wearing gloves in order to "better feel the vein". Though bare hands increase dexterity it is not worth the risk of transmitting infection.
- Sticking multiple times with one needle. If you fail to obtain a sample with your first stick you must use a new needle.
- Not properly cleaning the area. An alcohol cleansing agent should be used to properly clean the area of injection utilizing the cross hatch method and the area should be allowed to dry prior to needle insertion.
- Not capping needles. Butterfly syringes should be capped immediately upon withdraw from the patient.
- Not properly transferring blood to vacutainers. Blood should only be transferred to containers with shielded transfer devices.

Order of Blood Draws

Blood collection containers have specific additives to aid in running the tests. It is for this reason that a CBC cannot be placed in the same tube as a BMP for example. In order to prevent cross contamination of additives between tubes it is important that blood is drawn in a very specific order. Upon drawing the sample the vial should be inverted multiple times to insure proper mixing with the additive. For the most up to date information regarding the number of times for inversion please refer to the following website from Quest Diagnostics: http://goo.gl/u7CQ4q .

1. Blood Cultures (including tubes)
2. Light Blue
3. Red/Black
4. Red
5. Green
6. Lavender
7. Royal Blue
8. Gray
9. Yellow

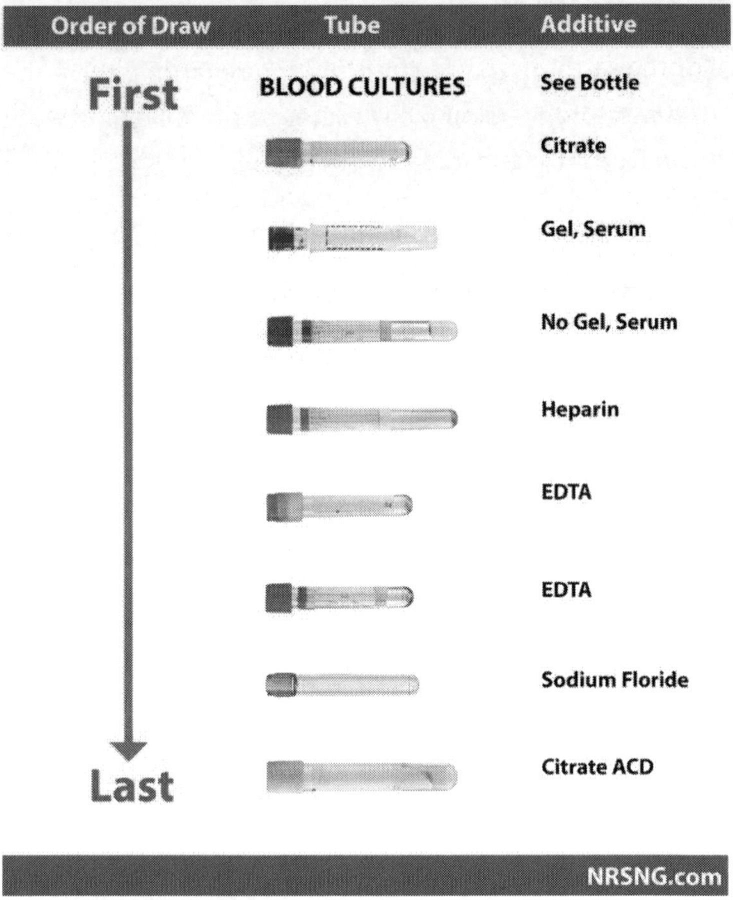

Methods of Blood Collection

There are two locations that blood sampling will come from in the adult patient; venous and arterial. The major differences seen on laboratory results will be demonstration in the fact that venous blood is oxygen deficient compared to arterial blood (pH, CO2, O2, Lactic acid). To appropriately assess a patient's respiratory status an arterial sample should be used. Otherwise it is appropriate to use venous or arterial blood (with exceptions for blood cultures) according to institutional guidelines. In critical care settings many patients will have central lines or arterial lines which provide direct access to blood samples. When direct access is not possible venous puncture technique can be used to obtain blood samples.

Prior to starting any laboratory draw it is important to pause fluid and TPN infusions (where clinically possible). Infusions like KPhos, 3%NaCl, and TPN solutions for example can have dramatic effects on laboratory data. TPN for example can elevate glucose readings up to and above 1000 mg/dL and excessive fluids can dilute venous blood and laboratory readings.

Venous Puncture

When obtaining a sample utilizing venous puncture the following supplies are needed:

1. Tourniquet
2. Butterfly needle
3. Gloves
4. Alcohol
5. Hubs
6. Blood collecting vial
7. Gauze pad
8. Tape

As with all procedures, two forms of patient identification should be provided prior to drawing blood. Insure that most recent orders have been viewed and maintain aseptic technique while drawing blood. While it can be tempting to aim for the larger veins within the antecubital fossa, patience is needed when searching for a vein that can be palpated with confidence. Depending on how much blood is needed for the sample a smaller distal vein may be used to draw the blood. The goal is to draw from a vein that is palpable.

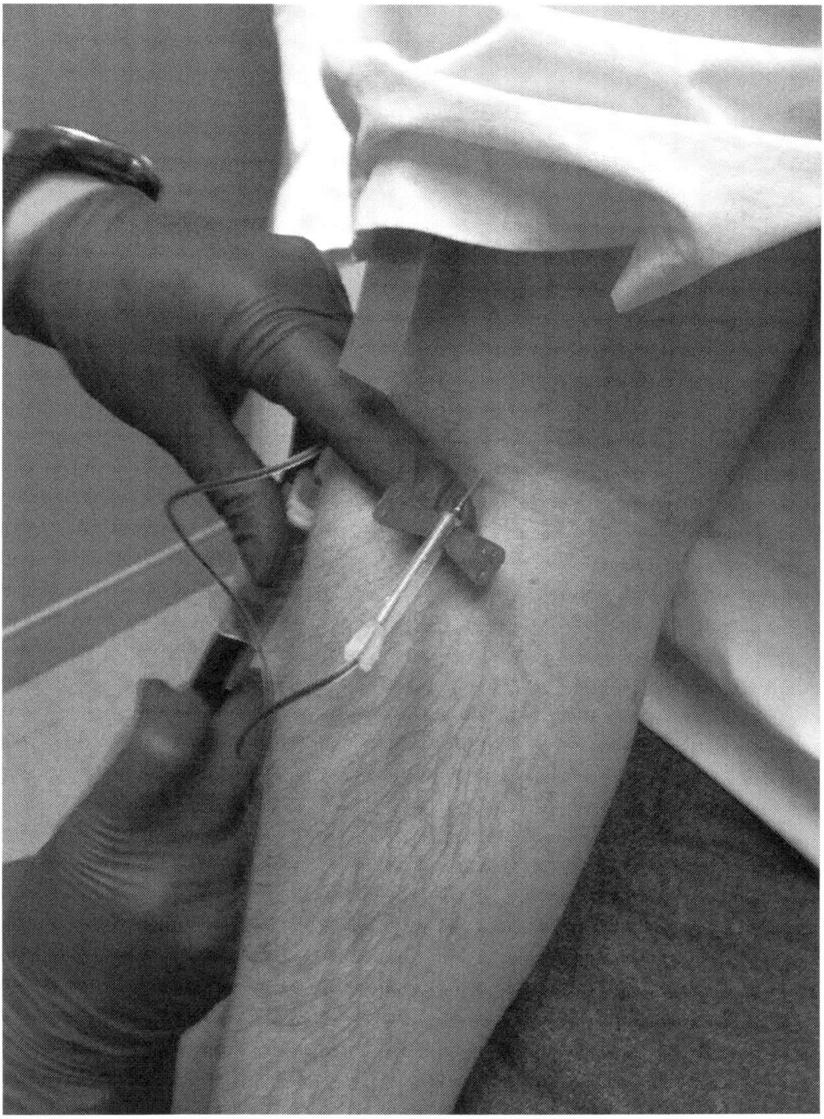

Flicker User: Walt Stoneburner

Arterial Line Draw

Laboratory samples including, obviously, ABGs can be drawn from arterial lines. With the use of a vamp system there is no need to draw a waste container as the blood drawn back into the vamp serves as the waste. This is helpful for a few reasons; it minimizes the amount of total blood drawn from the patient and can reduce the risk or severity of anemia suffered by patients during hospital stays, and it is slightly faster and easier on the nurse. If blood is being drawn through an art line that does not have a vamp system adequate waste must be drawn prior to drawing labs.

Central Lines and IVs

Blood sampling can be drawn from existing IVs and central lines utilizing aseptic technique. When drawing from IVs and central lines it is important that proper waste is drawn to avoid a contaminated sample. After blood draws are obtained it is important to flush the line to replace drawn fluid and to insure patent lines.

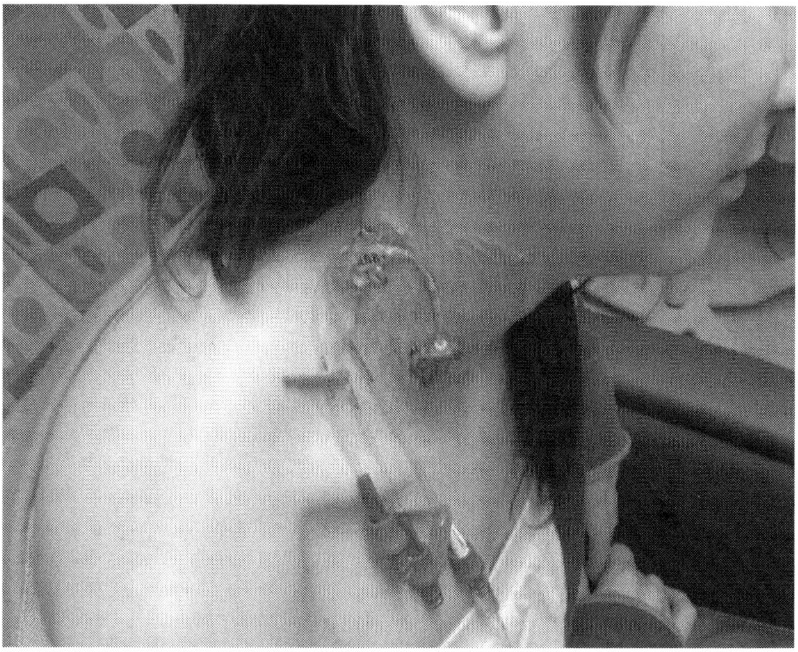

Special Considerations

When drawing any lab it is important to consider additional instructions regarding storage, transportation, and/or drawing technique. Lactic acid for example generally requires being transported to the laboratory on ice, creatinine clearance needs to be collected over 24 hours and refrigerated, blood cultures often have to be taken to the lab by hand. Lab labels, doctors orders, and laboratory orders should be reviewed closely to insure that all special considerations are being considered. Any questions or concerns should be referred to the lab or the ordering doctor.

Common Laboratory Tests and Values

Again, this is not a complete list of all possible lab tests. These charts include the most common lab values needed to know for the NCLEX®. Studying and knowing these values will prepare you for boards and to provide holistic care for patients.

I created a 4 page PDF download with all these lab values.

Get a FREE PDF download of these Lab Charts at NRSNG.com/Labs

Complete Blood Count (CBC) with Differential

Value	Abbreviation	Unit	Normal Range
Red Blood Cell	RBC	$x10^6$/ml	Male: 4.5 - 5.5 Female: 4.0 - 4.9
White Blood Cell	WBC	cells/mcL	4,500 - 10,000
Neutrophils			54 - 62%
Band Forms			3 - 5% (>8% = left shift)
Eosinophlis			1 - 3%
Basophils			0 - 0.75%
Lymphocytes			25 - 33%
Monocytes			3 - 7%
Platelets	PLT	cells/mcL	100,000 - 450,000
Hemoglobin	Hgb	g/dl	Male: 13.5 - 16.5 Female:

			12.0 - 15.0
Hematocrit	Hct	%	Male: 41 - 50 Female: 36 - 44
Mean Corpuscular Volume	MCV	fL	80 - 100
Red Cell Distribution Width	RDW		<14.5

Blood Chemistry (Basic Metabolic Panel) (BMP)			
Value	**Abbreviation**	**Unit**	**Normal Range**
Sodium	Na+	mEq/L	135 - 145
Potassium	K+	mEq/L	3.5 - 5.5
Chloride	Cl-	mEq/L	96 - 108
Glucose	Glu	mg/dL	70 - 115
Calcium	Ca^{2}+	mg/dL	8.4 - 10.2
Creatinine	Cr	mg/L	0.7-1.40
Blood Urea Nitrogen	BUN	mg/dL	7-20

Cholesterol Levels			
Value	**Abbreviation**	**Unit**	**Normal**
Cholesterol Total		mg/dL	<200
Low Density Lipoprotein	LDL	mg/dL	<70
High Density Lipoprotein	HDL	mg/dL	<60 optimal

Triglycerides		mg/dL	<150

Coagulation Studies			
Value	**Abbreviation**	**Unit**	**Normal**
Prothrombin Time	PT	Seconds	11 - 14
Partial Thromboplastin Time	PTT	Seconds	25 - 35
International Normalized Ratio	INR		0.8 - 1.2
Activated Partial Thromboplastin Time	aPTT		1.5 - 2.5

Arterial Blood Gas			
Value	**Abbreviation**	**Unit**	**Normal**
pH	pH		7.35 - 7.45
Partial Pressure of CO_2	pCO_2	mmHg	35 -45
Partial Pressure of O_2	pO_2	mmHg	80 - 100
Bicarbonate	HCO_3	mEq/L	22 - 26
Base Excess	BE	mEq/L	-2 - +2
Oxygen Saturation	SaO_2	%	95 - 100

Common Laboratory Tests			
Value	**Abbreviation**	**Unit**	**Normal**
Albumin	Alb	g/dL	3.5 - 6.0
Alkaline	Alk Phos	U/L	40 - 130

Phosphatase			
Aspartate Aminotransferase	AST	U/L	12 - 37
Alanine Aminotransferase	ALT	U/L	13 - 69
Activated Partial Thromboplastin Time	aPTT	seconds	25-39
Ammonia	NH_3	ug/dL	19 - 60
Amylase		U/L	0 - 130
Base Excess (Arterial)	BE	mEq/L	-2 - +2
Bicarbonate (Arterial)	HCO_3	mEq/L	22 - 26
Bilirubin, Direct (Conjugated)		mg/dL	0 - 0.2
Bilirubin, Total	T.billi	mg/dL	0.1 - 1.2
Blood Urea Nitrogen	BUN	mg/dL	7-20
Brain Type Natriuretic Peptide	BNP	pg/mL	<100
C-Reactive Protein	CRP	mg/L	<1.0
Calcium	Ca^2+	mg/dL	8.4 - 10.2
Chloride	Cl-	mEq/L	96 - 108
Cholesterol Total		mg/dL	<200
Creatinine	Cr	mg/dL	0.5 -1.2
Creatinine Clearance		$mL/min/1.73m^2$	85 - 125
Creatine Kinase	CK	U/L	55 - 170
Creatinine Kinase - MB	CK-MB	ng/mL	<2.40

D-Dimer	DDI	ng/mL	≤ 250
Erythrocyte Sedimentation Rate	ESR	mm/h	0 - 20
Ferritin		ng/mL	20-300
Folic Acid		ng/mL	2 - 20
Glomerular Filtration Rate	GFR	mL/min/1.73 m2	60
Glucose	Glu	mg/dL	70 - 115
Glucose Tolerance Test	GTT	mg/dL	Fasting: 60-100 1 hour: <200 2 hours: < 140
Glycosolated Hemoglobin	HgbA1c	% of total Hgb	5.6-7.5
Growth Hormone	GH	ng/mL	Male: <5 Female: < 10
Hematocrit	Hct	%	Male: 41 - 50 Female: 36 - 44
Hemoglobin	Hgb	g/dl	Male: 13.5 - 16.5 Female: 12.0 - 15.0
High Density Lipoprotein	HDL	mg/dL	<60 optimal
Homocysteine		mg/L	0.54 - 2.3

International Normalized Ratio	INR		0.8 - 1.2
Iron	Fe	ug/dL	50-175
Lactate Dehydrogenase	LDH	U/L	88-230
Lactic Acid		mEq/L	Venous Blood: 0.5-2.2 Arterial Blood: 0.5-1.6
Lipase		U/L	23 - 300
Low Density Lipoprotein	LDL	mg/dL	<70
Magnesium	Mg	mg/dL	1.6 – 2.6
Mean Corpuscular Volume	MCV	fL	80 - 100
Myoglobin	MB	ng/mL	5 – 70
Osmolality, Serum		mOSM/kg	261-280
Oxygen Saturation (Arterial)	SaO_2	%	95 - 100
Partial Pressure of (Arterial) CO_2	pCO_2	mmHg	35 -40
Partial Pressure of (Arterial) O_2	pO_2	mmHg	80 - 100
Partial Thromboplastin Time	PTT	Seconds	25 - 35
pH (arterial)	pH		7.35 - 7.45
Phosphorus	PO_4	mg/dL	3.0-4.5

(phosphate)			
Platelets	PLT	cells/mcL	100,000 - 450,000
Potassium	K+	mEq/L	3.5 - 5.5
Prealbumin	PAB	mg/dL	19-38
Prostate Specific Antigen	PSA	ng/mL	Male: < 4 Female: < 0.5
Protein (total)	Prot	g/dL	6-8
Prothrombin Time	PT	Seconds	11 - 14
Red Blood Cell	RBC	$x10^6$/cells/mm^3	Male: 4.5 - 5.5 Female: 4.0 - 4.9
Red Cell Distribution Width	RDW		<14.5
Sodium	Na+	mEq/L	135 - 145
Triglycerides	TG	mg/dL	<150
Total Iron Binding Capacity	TIBC	ug/dL	250-460
Troponin I	cTnI	ng/mL	<0.035
White Blood Cell	WBC	cells/mcL	4,500 - 10,000

Get a FREE PDF download of these Lab Charts at NRSNG.com/Labs

Explanation of Lab Values

Albumin

Normal

3.5 - 6.0 g/dL

Indications

evaluation of chronic illness, liver disease, or nutritional status

Description

Albumin is a transport protein in the blood. It helps maintain the oncotic pressure of the blood. Albumin levels will drop if synthesis is slowed, protein intake is inadequate, or there are increased losses. Albumin has a long half life, however, so levels are not a good indicator of acute illness.

What would cause increased levels?

dehydration, hyper infusion of albumin

What would cause decreased levels?

inadequate intake, liver disease, inflammation, chronic disease, losses (fistula, hemorrhage, kidney disease, burns), over hydration, Increased catabolism, congestive heart failure

Alkaline Phosphatase

Normal

40-130 U/L

Indications

identifying hepatobiliary disease, malignancies, bone disease, bone damage in renal patients; useful in evaluating bone growth in children.

Description

Alkaline phosphatase (ALP) is located in several places in the body: liver, intestines, biliary tract, bones, placenta. Different isoenzymes of ALP can be used to determine different disorders: liver, bone, intestine, certain cancers. It can also be used to determine bone turnover in postmenopausal women.

What would cause increased levels?

liver disease, bone disease, pregnancy, amyloidosis, lung cancer, pancreatic cancer, congestive heart failure, ulcerative colitis, Hodgkin's disease, chronic renal failure, sarcoidosis

What would cause decreased levels?

hypophophatasia, anemia, kwashiorkor, cretinism, hypothyroidism, zinc or magnesium deficiency, scurvy

Aspartate Aminotransferase

Normal

12-37 U/L

Indications

monitor progression of liver disease, and response to treatments.

Description

Aspartate aminotranferase (AST) is an enzyme primarily found in liver and heart cells. To a smaller extent it is also found in pancreas, kidneys, skeletal muscle, and brain.

What would cause increased levels?

Liver disease, shock, pancreatitis, CHF, Liver Cancer, dermatomyositis, muscular dystrophy, biliary tract obstruction

What would cause decreased levels?

CVA, delirium tremens, pericarditis, cirrhosis, hemolytic anemia

Alanine Aminotransferase

Normal

13 – 69 U/L

Indications

monitoring progression of liver disease or liver damage. It can also aid in monitoring response to treatments

Description

ALT is an enzyme made in the liver. This enzyme is found in highest concentrations in the liver , but is found to lesser extent in heart, skeletal muscle and kidney. Damage to the liver results in a significant increase in this enzyme.

What would cause increased levels?

cirrhosis, muscle damage, preeclampsia, biliary tract obstruction, burns, Pancreatitis, long-term alcohol abuse, Liver Cancer, muscular dystrophy, MI, myositis, shock, infections mononucleosis

What would cause decreased levels?

pyridoxal phosphate deficiency

Activated Partial Thromboplastin Time

Normal

25-39 seconds

Indications

identifying congenital deficiencies in clotting; monitoring effects of liver disease, protein deficiency, fat malabsorption on clotting.

Description

APPT is a test that measures the amount of time it takes for a fibrin clot to form after reagents have been added to the specimen. It is useful in diagnosis clotting disorders. In conjunction with PT it can be used to differentiate the specific factor that may be missing.

What would cause increased levels?

vitamin K deficiency, DIC, patients on hemodialysis, afibrinogenemia, polycythemia, liver disease, Von Willebrand disease.

What would cause decreased levels?

N/A

Ammonia

Normal

19-60 µg/dL

Indications

identifying liver disease, monitoring hepatic encephalopathy, and evaluating effectiveness of treatment.

Description

Ammonia is a byproduct created when protein is broken down. Ammonia is converted into urea in the liver, and urea is excreted by the kidneys. During liver disease ammonia levels rise and can have a negative effect on the brain.

What would cause increased levels?

gastrointestinal hemorrhage, liver failure, hepatic coma, Reye's syndrome, TPN

What would cause decreased levels?

N/A

Amylase

Normal

0-130 U/L

Indications

diagnosing pancreatitis, macroamylasemia, pancreatic duct obstruction, trauma to pancreas.

Description

Amylase is made in the pancreas. It is an enzyme that breaks down carbohydrate to allow our body to absorb it. Monitoring amylase levels can identify problems with the pancreas

What would cause increased levels?

alcoholism, pancreatitis, DKA, peritonitis, abdominal trauma, pancreatic cancer, duodenal obstruction, gastric resection, mumps, pancreatic cyst

What would cause decreased levels?

cystic fibrosis, liver disease, pancreatic insufficiency, pancreatectomy

Base Excess

Normal

-2 - +2 mEq/L

Indications

identifying metabolic acidosis and alkalosis

Description

Base excess represents the amount of anions in the blood that can help buffer against changes in pH. Base excess is altered when bicarbonate levels are either high or low. If base excess is low or high it indicates a metabolic cause of acidosis or alkalosis. Negative base excess indicates metabolic acidosis.

What would cause increased levels?

metabolic alkalosis (alkali ingestion, gastric suctioning, low potassium, Cushing's disease, diuresis, diarrhea, vomiting)

What would cause decreased levels?

Metabolic acidosis (DKA, Addison's disease, Wilson's disease, renal failure, diarrhea, fistula, increased acid intake)

Bicarbonate

Normal

22-26 mEq

Indications

differentiate between metabolic and respiratory causes of pH imbalances.

Description

Bicarbonate is a base and anion that helps to neutralize acids in the blood. Bicarbonate needs to be 20 times carbonic acid to maintain balance in the blood. Bicarbonate HCO_3^- levels can either be measured or determined using carbon dioxide levels

What would cause increased levels?

anoxia, respiratory acidosis, metabolic alkalosis

What would cause decreased levels?

hypocapnia, respiratory alkalosis, metabolic acidosis

Direct Bilirubin

Normal

0-0.2 mg/dL

Indications

useful when used in correlation with total bilirubin, used to determine amount of unconjugated bilirubin, an elevated unconjugated bilirubin indicates a problem with the liver

Description

Bilirubin is a byproduct of red blood cell breakdown. Bilirubin is transported to the liver where it is conjugated. It then goes to the intestines to be excreted. Direct bilirubin is a measure of conjugated bilirubin. If you subtract direct bilirubin from total bilirubin you can determine the amount of unconjugated bilirubin. If unconjugated bilirubin is elevated that is specific to liver disease

What would cause increased levels?

elevated destruction of red blood cells, liver problems

What would cause decreased levels?

N/A

Total Bilirubin

Normal

0.1 - 1.2 mg/dL

Indications

identifying liver disease, obstructive jaundice, biliary disease, newborn jaundice, and effectiveness of treatment.

Description

One of the by-products of red blood cell breakdown is bilirubin. Bilirubin is made in the bone marrow, liver, or spleen and is transported by albumin to the liver. In the liver bilirubin is conjugated. In the small intestine conjugated bilirubin is eventually excreted in the feces as urobilin. Excess bilirubin causes a yellowing of the skin and the whites of the eyes called jaundice.

What would cause increased levels?

post-blood transfusions, hematoma, newborn jaundice, pernicious anemia, hepatic jaundice, liver tumors, biliary obstruction, Gilbert's disease, alcoholism, cholesytitis, cholangitis, cirrhosis, hepatitis, Mono, hypothyroidism, breast milk jaundice.

What would cause decreased levels?

N/A

Blood Urea Nitrogen

Normal

7-20 mg/dL

Indications

identify liver problems, renal problems, hydration status, tumor lysis; evaluate effects of drugs on liver or kidney; monitor effectiveness of hemodialysis

Description

When protein is broken down ammonia is formed. Ammonia is converted to urea in the liver and is eventually excreted in the kidneys. Blood urea nitrogen (BUN) measures the amount of urea in the blood.

What would cause increased levels?

renal failure, CHF, kidney disease, DM, excessive protein intake, GI bleed, shock, dehydration, ketoacidosis, neoplasm, urinary tract obstruction.

What would cause decreased levels?

liver failure, over-hydration, inadequate protein intake, pregnancy

Brain Type Natriuretic Peptide

Normal

<100 pg/mL

Indications

identify congestive heart failure, effectiveness of treatment, or severity of disease.

Description

Brain natriuretic peptide (BNP) is a hormone. It is made by the heart and indicates how hard the heart is working. When levels are increased it indicates that the heart is working too hard

What would cause increased levels?

CHF

What would cause decreased levels?

N/A

C-Reactive Protein

Normal

<1.0 mg/L

Indications

differentiate between appendicitis vs pelvic inflammatory disease, Crohn's vs ulcerative colitis, rheumatoid arthritis and lupus (SLE - systemic lupus erythematosus); monitor or identify inflammation in the body, evaluate coronary artery disease.

Description

C-reactive protein (CRP) is made in the liver in response to inflammation. CRP helps practitioners identify inflammation and when it has resolved. CRP is a good indicator because it increases quickly in the inflammatory response, and drops when inflammation resolves.

What would cause increased levels?

bacterial infection, Crohn's disease, inflammatory bowel disease, lupus, rheumatoid arthritis, pregnancy, myocardial infarction.

What would cause decreased levels?

N/A

Calcium

Normal

8.4-10.2 mg/dL

Indications

identify problems with parathyroid, diseases that affect bone, effectiveness of treatments.

Description

Calcium (Ca^+) is a positive ion in the body. The parathyroid gland and Vitamin D are responsible for Calcium regulation in the body. Calcium is primarily located in bone and teeth, but is also found in the blood and inside cells. Other than a major component of bone, Calcium also participates in muscle contraction. In the blood about 45% of Calcium travels in ion form, 40% is bound to proteins like albumin, 15% bound to anions like bicarbonate, lactate, etc. When albumin levels are low, Calcium levels will appear lower. Calcium has an important relationship with Phosphorus: they are inversely proportional.

What would cause increased levels?

cancers (lymphoma, leukemia, bone), acidosis, dehydration, excess Ca intake, hyperparathyroidism, pheochromocytoma, polycythemia vera, renal transplant, sarcoidosis, vitamin D toxicity.

What would cause decreased levels?

malnutrition, cirrhosis, hypoparathyroidism, alkalosis, chronic renal failure, Magnesium deficiency, hypoalbunemia, hyperphosphatemia, malabsorption, alcoholism, osteomalacia, Vitamin D deficiency.

Chloride

Normal

97-107 mEq/L

Indications

identify different types of acidosis.

Description

Chloride (Cl^-) is an anion found in the blood. Sodium and chloride help maintain oncotic pressure and water balance in the body. Chloride is inversely related to bicarbonate levels in the blood. Chloride is a part of HCL which is utilized in the stomach to breakdown food. When red blood cells take up CO_2 they take up chloride as well. The negative ion bicarbonate then leaves the red blood cell so that the electrical charge is maintained. Extra chloride is excreted into the urine by the kidneys.

What would cause increased levels?

dehydration, acute renal failure, Cushing's disease, hyperparathyroidism, metabolic acidosis, respiratory alkalosis.

What would cause decreased levels?

congestive heart failure, overhydration, water intoxication, burns, metabolic alkalosis, Addison's disease, salt-losing nephritis, excessive sweating, diarrhea, vomiting, fistula.

Cholesterol

Normal

<200 mg/dL

Indications

determine risk of cardiovascular disease; diagnose nephrotic disease, hepatic disease, pancreatitis; gauge response to treatment.

Description

Cholesterol (Chol) is a lipid in the body. It is a part of cell membranes, a precursor for vitamin D, steroids, bile acids. Cholesterol is primarily synthesized in the liver and intestines. It is transported via lipoproteins. There are multiple types of lipoproteins and they each have slightly different functions: high-density lipoprotein (HDL), low-density lipoprotein, LDL, very low-density lipoprotein (VLDL).

What would cause increased levels?

tangier disease, myeloma, burns, pernicious anemia, thalassemia, waldensrom's macroglobulinemia, chronic myelocytic leukemia, malabsorbtion, malnutrition, liver disease, polycythemia vera, chronic obstructive pulmonary disease, hyperthyroidism, myeloma

What would cause decreased levels?

Gout, Obesity, high fat diet, pregnancy, nephrotic syndrome, werner's syndrome, von Gierke disease, alcoholism, anorexia, ischemic heart disease, acute intermittent porphyria, pancreatic malignancy

Creatinine

Normal

0.5-1.2 mg/dL

Indications

identify muscular disorders or renal disease.

Description

Creatinine is a byproduct of creatine metabolism, and it is excreted in the kidneys. Creatinine is created in proportion to muscle mass and usually stays stable.

What would cause increased levels?

gigantism, dehydration, shock, renal disease, rhabdomyolysis, acromegaly, CHF, hyperparathyroidism

What would cause decreased levels?

loss of muscle mass, inadequate protein intake, pregnancy, liver disease, muscular dystrophy

Creatinine Clearance

Normal

Male: 97 to 137 ml/min
Female: 88 to 128 ml/min

Indications

used to determine kidney damage in renal disease, glomerular function, effectiveness of treatment.

Description

Creatinine is a byproduct of creatine metabolism, and it is excreted in the kidneys. Creatinine is created in proportion to muscle mass and usually stays stable. Urine and blood levels are compared to determine creatinine clearance from the blood.

What would cause increased levels?

DM, exercise, renal disease, tuberculosis, acromegaly, gigantism, congestive heart failure, high protein diet, polycystic kidney disease, dehydration, infections, hypothyroidism.

What would cause decreased levels?

glomerulonephritis, paralysis, vegetarian diet, anemia, leukemia, shock, muscle wasting, hyperparathyroidism, polycystic kidney disease

Creatine Kinase

Normal

55 - 170 U/L

Indications

diagnose acute MI, ischemia, dermatomyosis, muscular dystrophy; evaluate success of treatment

Description

Creatine Kinase enzyme is found in heart and skeletal muscle and to a lesser extent brain. When damage is done to these types of tissue CK is released into the blood. There are three isoenzymes, and depending on which one is elevated this lab value can help one determine timing, location, extent of damage. The three isoenzymes are CK-MB (cardiac), CK-MM (skeletal), and CK-BB (brain).

What would cause increased levels?

alcoholism, brain infarction, congestive heart failure, delirium tremens, dermatomyositis, head injury hypothyroidism, hypoxic shock, infectious disease, gastrointestinal tract infection, loss of blood supply to muscle, muscular dystrophy, myocardial infarction, myocarditis, neoplasms of the prostate, bladder of GI tract, polymyositis, pregnancy, hypothermia, pulmonary edema, pulmonary embolism, reye's sydrome, rhabdomyolysis, surgery, tachycardia, tetanus, trauma.

What would cause decreased levels?

small stature, sedentary lifestyle

Creatine Kinase -MB

Normal

< 2.40 ng/mL

Indications

diagnose acute MI, identify ischemia

Description

Creatine Kinase enzyme is found in heart and skeletal muscle and to a lesser extent brain. When damage is done to these types of tissue CK is released into the blood. There are three isoenzymes, and depending on which one is elevated this lab value can help one determine timing, location, extent of damage. The three isoenzymes are CK-MB (cardiac), CK-MM (skeletal), and CK-BB (brain). If CK-MB is elevated 3 times more than CK this indicates damage to heart muscle

What would cause increased levels?

damage to the heart including ischemia, surgery, trauma, inflammation; kidney failure

What would cause decreased levels?

n/a

D-Dimer

Normal

≤ 250 ng/mL

Indications

Identify DIC and rule out pulmonary embolism, DVT, or stroke.

Description

D-dimer is a compound formed when two identical fibrin molecules combine. Cross-linkages do not occur between fibrinogen molecules. D-dimer levels are elevated in the setting of clot breakdown, but will be even higher in the setting of DIC

What would cause increased levels?

surgery, trauma, infection, liver disease, cancer, pregnancy, DVT, DIC, cardiac disease

What would cause decreased levels?

N/A

Erythrocyte Sedimentation Rate

Normal

0-20 mm/h

Indications

identifies inflammation which assists in diagnosing cancer, infection, and autoimmune diseases.

Description

The erythrocyte sedimentation rate (ESR) test measures sedimentation of red blood cells. The inflammatory process affects proteins in the blood which causes red blood cells to stick together and settle out of liquid. Normal blood has very little settling, but during the inflammatory process the ESR is elevated.

What would cause increased levels?

myocardial infarction, anemia, cancers, systemic lupus erythromatosus, Crohn's disease, endocarditis, infection, lymphoma, multiple myeloma, nephritis, pregnancy, pulmonary embolism, rheumatoid arthritis, tuberculosis.

What would cause decreased levels?

CHF, sickle cell anemia, polycythemia

Ferritin

Normal

20-300 ng/mL

Indications

diagnosing iron-deficiency anemia or hemochromatosis, monitor iron levels during pregnancy

Description

Ferritin is the storage form of Iron. Some is stored in body tissue, some circulates in the blood. It is formed in the liver spleen and bone marrow. Ferritin in the blood is usually proportional to stored ferritin. Ferritin is a more sensitive and specific test for identifying iron-deficiency anemia, however, it is usually measured in conjunction with total iron binding capacity and iron.

What would cause increased levels?

inflammation, breast cancer, hemolytic anemia, fasting, hemochromatosis, liver disease, hyperthyroidism, alcoholism, Hodgkin's disease, infection, leukemia

What would cause decreased levels?

dialysis, iron-deficiency anemia

Folic Acid

Normal

2 - 20 ng/mL

Indications

diagnosis of megaloblastic anemia, monitor effects of long-term total parenteral nutrition, identify folate deficiency

Description

Folate is an essential water soluble vitamin. It is stored in the liver and is an important part of RBC and WBC function, DNA replication, and cell division.

What would cause increased levels?

Vitamin B12 deficiency, excess folate intake, pernicious anemia

What would cause decreased levels?

malnutrition, hemolytic anemias, scurvy, liver disease, Crohn's disease, megaloblastic anemia, neoplasm, alcoholism, pregnancy, sideroblastic anemias, ulcerative colitis, whipple's disease.

Glomerular Filtration Rate

Normal

60 mL/min/1.73 m2

Indications

indicator of kidney disease, useful tool in evaluating the extent of kidney damage.

Description

Glomerular filtration rate (GFR) is an estimate of blood flow through the kidneys. There are different equations used to estimate the GFR. A GFR <60 ml mL/min/1.73 m2 for over 3 months indicates chronic kidney disease. A GFR < 15 mL/min/1.73 m2 indicates kidney failure.

What would cause increased levels?

N/A

What would cause decreased levels?

kidney disease, kidney failure

Glucose

Normal

70-115 mg/dL

Indications

diagnosis of insulinemia, identifying hypoglycemia, assist in diagnosing diabetes, monitor treatments for diabetes

Description

Glucose is a sugar molecule that is a component of carbohydrates. In the body sugar is stored as glycogen in liver and muscle. Glucose is a very important source of energy in the body. The pancreas helps regulate levels of glucose in the blood so that levels are never too high or too low. Glucose levels naturally rise after meals with the intake of carbohydrates.

What would cause increased levels?

stress (physical and emotional), pancreatitis, stroke, Cushing's syndrome, DM, hemochromatosis, liver disease, myocardial infarction, pancreatic adenoma, renal disease, shock, trauma, strenuous exercise, Vitamin B1 deficiency

What would cause decreased levels?

malabsorption syndromes, alcohol ingestion, glucagon deficiency, von Gierke disease, hypothyroidism, Addison's disease, maple syrup urine disease, starvation, post-gastrectomy,

Glucose Tolerance Test

Normal

Fasting: 60-100 mg/dL
1 hour: <200 mg/dL
2 hours: < 140 mg/dL

Indications

identify impaired glucose metabolism

Description

The glucose tolerance test (GTT) is a measure of glucose metabolism after a specific amount of glucose intake. A fasting blood sugar is taken and then a 75 gram carbohydrate drink is taken. Blood sugars are measured 1 hour, 2 hour, and 3 hour post-prandial. Blood sugars over 126 mg/dL fasting or >200 mg/dL after 2 hours indicate a problem in glucose metabolism.

What would cause increased levels?

elevated numbers indicate impaired glucose metabolism

What would cause decreased levels?

N/A

Glycosylated Hemoglobin

Normal

5.6-7.5 % of total hgb

Indications

assess control of blood sugars over a several month time frame

Description

Glycosylated hemoglobin (Hgb A1c) is the combination of sugar in the blood (glucose) and hemoglobin. When glucose is elevated in the blood the amount of glycosylated hemoglobin increases proportionally. A red blood cells lifespan is about 4 months, so you can get an idea of blood sugar control over the last several months.

What would cause increased levels?

DM

What would cause decreased levels?

renal failure, blood loss, pregnancy, hemolytic anemia.

Growth Hormone

Normal

Male: <5 ng/mL
Female: < 10 ng/mL

Indications

diagnosing acromegaly, dwarfism, or gigantism.

Description

Growth hormone is secreted by the anterior pituitary. Growth hormone helps regulate sleep and growth throughout childhood. Growth hormone stimulates protein production and lipid and glucose metabolism.

What would cause increased levels?

cirrhosis, acromegaly, Exercise, hyperpituitarism, gigantism, malnutrition, anorexia nervosa, diabetes, renal failure, stress

What would cause decreased levels?

dwarfism, hypopituitarism

Hematocrit

Normal

Male: 41 - 50%
Female: 36 - 44%

Indications

identify anemia, bleeding, bleeding disorder, fluid imbalances.

Description

Hematocrit is the percentage of the blood that is made up of packed red blood cells. A hematocrit level of 40% indicates that there are 40 mL packed red blood cells in 100mL of blood.

What would cause increased levels?

erythrocytosis, polycythemia, shock, dehydration

What would cause decreased levels?

anemia, blood loss, bone marrow hyperplasia, severe burns,

Hemoglobin

Normal

Male: 13.5 - 16.5 g/dL
Female: 12.0 - 15.0 g/dL

Indications

identify bleeding disorders, anemia, blood loss,

Description

Hemoglobin is the main protein in red blood cells. It binds to and transports oxygen in the blood, and can also carry carbon dioxide. Hemoglobin is an iron containing compound, And iron-deficiency can affect hemoglobin's ability to carry oxygen.

What would cause increased levels?

burns, COPD, CHF, dehydration, eryhrocytosis, high altitudes, polycythemia vera

What would cause decreased levels?

hemolytic disorders, nutrition deficiency, fluid retention, anemias, Hodgkin's disease, hemorrhage, leukemia, carcinoma, lymphoma, pregnancy

High Density Lipoprotein

Normal

<60 optimal mg/dL

Indications

HDL cholesterol is beneficial, and lower levels indicate increased risk for heart disease.

Description

Cholesterol is transported via lipoproteins. There are multiple types of lipoproteins and they each have slightly different functions: high-density lipoprotein (HDL), low-density lipoprotein, LDL, very low-density lipoprotein (VLDL). HDL cholesterol is considered the good cholesterol as it travels through the blood picking up extra cholesterol and taking it back to the liver.

What would cause increased levels?

exercise, mono- and poly- unsaturated fats

What would cause decreased levels?

smoking, high saturated and trans fat diet, excess body weight

Homocysteine

Normal

0.54 - 2.3 mg/L

Indications

identify enzyme deficiencies that cause homocystinuria, evaluate risk of cardiovascular disease or venous thrombosis.

Description

Homocysteine is an amino acid in the body that can be synthesized from the amino acid methionine. Homocysteine required vitamin B12 and Folate to break it down. Excess homocysteine can damage blood vessels, impact clotting, and increase risk of plaque formation.

What would cause increased levels?

chronic renal failure, folic acid deficiency, homocystinuria, Vitamin B12 deficiency, coronary artery disease.

What would cause decreased levels?

N/A

International Normalized Ratio

Normal

0.8 - 1.2

Indications

evaluate therapeutic doses of anticoagulants, identify patients at higher risk for bleeding, identify cause of bleeding, and deficiencies

Description

International normalized ratio (INR) takes results from a prothrombin time test and standardizes it regardless of collection method.

What would cause increased levels?

disseminated intravascular coagulation, hereditary factors, liver disease, vitamin k deficiency, SLE, drug therapy,

What would cause decreased levels?

enteritis, ovarian hyperfunction

Iron

Normal

50-175 ug/dL

Indications

identify blood loss, hemochromatosis, malabsorption of iron, iron overload, type of anemia, thalassemia, or sideroblastic anemia

Description

Iron is an element that is an important component of hemoglobin in red blood cells. Hemoglobin transports oxygen from the lungs to all the cells of the body. Most of the iron in the body is in hemoglobin, but some iron is in myoglobin and some is stored in the liver, bone marrow, and spleen. The storage form of iron is ferritin. Iron is transported in the blood by a protein called transferrin.

What would cause increased levels?

hemolytic anemia, iron poisoning, sideroblastic anemia, acute leukemia, Vitamin B6 deficiency acute liver disease, hemochromatosis, aplastic anemia, nephritis, thalassemia, pernicious anemia, lead toxicity

What would cause decreased levels?

infection, carcinoma, blood loss, hypothyroidism, iron-deficiency anemia, nephrosis, protein malnutrition

Lactic Acid

Normal

0.3 -2.6 mMol/L

Indications

determine cause of acidosis, evaluate tissue oxygenation

Description

Lactate is a byproduct of carbohydrate metabolism. Lactate is broken down by the liver. During intense exercise pyruvate is converted to lactate to provide a little extra energy when there is not enough oxygen present. If the liver doesn't properly breakdown lactate that can lead to increased levels.

What would cause increased levels?

DM, heart failure, hemorrhage, excess alcohol consumption, lactic acidosis, pulmonary embolism, reye's syndrome, shock, strenuous exercise.

What would cause decreased levels?

N/A

Lipase

Normal

23 - 300 U/L

Indications

diagnose pancreatitis, diagnose pancreatic cancer

Description

Lipase is an enzyme created in the pancreas. It travels to the intestines where it aids in the breakdown of fats. If damage occurs to certain parts of the pancreas lipase is released into the bloodstream.

What would cause increased levels?

cholecystitis, pancreatic duct obstruction, pancreatic cyst, pseudocyst, pancreatic inflammation, pancreatitis, renal failure.

What would cause decreased levels?

N/A

Low Density Lipoprotein

Normal

<70 mg/dL

Indications

Useful in determining risk of cardiovascular disease.

Description

Cholesterol is transported via lipoproteins. There are multiple types of lipoproteins and they each have slightly different functions: high-density lipoprotein (HDL), low-density lipoprotein, LDL, very low-density lipoprotein (VLDL).

What would cause increased levels?

diet high in saturated fats

What would cause decreased levels?

regular physical activity

Magnesium

Normal

1.6 – 2.6 mg/dL

Indications

monitor renal failure, chronic alcoholism, monitor cardiac arrhythmias,

Description

Magnesium is a cation necessary for protein synthesis, nucleic acid synthesis, muscle contraction, ADP (adenosine diphosphate) use, nerve impulse conduction, and blood clotting. Magnesium affects the absorption of sodium, calcium, phosphorus, potassium.

What would cause increased levels?

Addison's disease, adrenocorticol insufficiency, dehydration, diabetic acidosis, hypothyroidism, SLE, multiple myeloma, overuse of antacids, renal insufficiency, tissue trauma

What would cause decreased levels?

alcoholism, diabetic acidosis, glomerulonephritis, hemodialysis, hypercalcemia, hypoparathyroidism, inadequate Mg intake, malabsorption, pancreatitis, pregnancy, diarrhea

Mean corpuscular volume

Normal

80-100 fl

Indications

assist in anemia diagnosis, identify hematologic disorders

Description

Mean corpuscular volume (MCV) is the average of the volume of red blood cells. It is helpful in differentiating between different types of anemia.

What would cause increased levels?

alcoholism, antimetabolite therapy, liver disease, pernicious anemia, Vitamin B12 anemia, folate anemia

What would cause decreased levels?

iron-deficiency anemia, thalassemia

Myoglobin

Normal

5-70 ng/mL

Indications

identifying damage from a MI or skeletal muscle damage.

Description

Myoglobin is a protein in skeletal and cardiac muscle that binds oxygen. When damage is done to heart and skeletal muscle, myoglobin is released into the blood.

What would cause increased levels?

rhabdomyolysis, heart surgery, exercise, cocaine use, MI, muscular dystrophy, shock, renal failure

What would cause decreased levels?

myasthenia gravis, rheumatoid arthritis

Osmolality

Normal

261 – 280 mOsm/kg

Indications

monitor electrolyte balance and acid-base balance, monitor hydration, evaluate function of antidiuretic hormone.

Description

Osmolality is a measure of the particles in solution. The size, shape, and charge of the particles do not impact the osmolality

What would cause increased levels?

dehydration, azotemia, hypercalcemia, diabetic ketoacidosis, hypernatremia, diabetes insipidus

What would cause decreased levels?

adrenocorticoid insufficiency, hyponatremia, syndrome of inappropriate antidiuretic hormone

Oxygen Saturation SaO2

Normal

95 - 100%

Indications

as part of the ABG to determine respiratory status

Description

Oxygen is transported in the blood in two ways. Oxygen dissolved in blood plasma (pO_2) and oxygen bound to hemoglobin (SaO_2). About 97% of oxygen is bound to hemoglobin while 3% is dissolved in plasma. There is a relationship between saturation and partial pressure referred to the oxyhemoglobin dissociation curve. SaO_2 of about 90% is associated with PO_2 of about 60 mmHg.

Partial Pressure of CO_2

Normal

35 - 45 mmHg

Indications

part of the ABG reflects the amount of CO_2 dissolved in the blood

Description

pCO_2 is an indirect measure of gas exchange within the lungs.

What would cause increased levels?

CO_2 retention: pulmonary edema, COPD

What would cause decreased levels?

hyperventilation, hypoxia, anxiety, pregnancy, pulmonary embolism

Partial Pressure of O2

Normal

80 - 100 mmHg

Indications

part of an ABG to determine respiratory status

Description

Oxygen is transported in the blood in two ways. Oxygen dissolved in blood plasma (pO_2) and oxygen bound to hemoglobin (SaO_2). About 97% of oxygen is bound to hemoglobin while 3% is dissolved in plasma. There is a relationship between saturation and partial pressure referred to the oxyhemoglobin dissociation curve. SaO_2 of about 90% is associated with PO_2 of about 60 mmHg

What would cause increased levels?

↑ O_2 in inhaled air, polycythemia

What would cause decreased levels?

↓O_2 in inhaled air, anemia, cardiac decompensation, COPD, restrictive pulmonary disease, hypoventilation

Partial Thromboplastin Time

Normal

25 - 35 seconds

Indications

detection of coagulation disorders, evaluate response to anticoagulation medication, preoperative assessment

Description

Partial Thromboplastin Time (PTT) evaluates the function of factors XII, XI, IX, VII, V, X, II, and I, represents the amount of time required for a fibrin clot to form

What would cause increased levels?

DIC, factor deficiencies, liver disease, vitamin K deficiency, polycythemia, dialysis, Von Willebrand's disease

What would cause decreased levels?

N/A

pH (partial pressure of Hydrogen ion)

Normal

7.35 - 7.45

Description

reflects the amount of free H+ ions in the body

What would cause increased levels?

Metabolic alkalosis - suctioning, potassium depletion, diarrhea, vomiting

Respiratory alkalosis - stimulation of the respiratory center, hyperventilation, fever

What would cause decreased levels?

Metabolic acidosis- DKA, decreased excretion of H+, increased acid intake

Respiratory acidosis - asthma, bronchoconstriction, emphysema, pneumonia

Phosphorus

Normal

3.0-4.5 mg/dL

Indications

diagnosing hyperparathyroidism, evaluation of renal failure

Description

Phosphorus is a major intracellular anion playing a vital role in cellular metabolism. it makes up the phospholipid bilayer of the cell membrane, and is crucial in the formation of bones and teeth. Calcium and phosphorus share an inverse relationship

What would cause increased levels?

excess vitamin D, DKA, lactic acidosis, renal failure (excreted by kidneys), pulmonary embolism, respiratory acidosis, hypocalcemia, acromegaly

What would cause decreased levels?

hyperalimentation, hyperinsulinism, hyperparathyroidism, hypokalemia, hypercalcemia, alkalosis, vomiting and diarrhea, malnutrition, osteomalacia

Platelets

Normal

100,000 - 450,000 cells/mcL

Indications

determine clotting vs bleeding disorders, part of a basic screening exam

Description

platelets play a role in coagulation, hemostasis, and thrombus formation. Platelets are the smallest blood cell, damaged vessels send out signals that result in platelets traveling to the area and becoming "active".

What would cause increased levels?

infection, bone marrow disorders (polycythemia vera), RA, malignancy, cirrhosis, pancreatitis, trauma

What would cause decreased levels?

aplastic anemia, alcoholism, medication, inherited, carcinoma, lymphoma, uremia, hemorrhage, DIC, bacterial infection, Idiopathic thrombocytopenic purpura, radiation, dialysis

Potassium

Normal

3.5 - 5.5 mEq/L

Indications

evaluate electrolyte imbalances, useful in evaluating cardiac arrhythmias, useful when patient is receiving diuretic therapy, useful with acidotic patients

Description

potassium is the most abundant intracellular cation and plays a vital role in the transmission of electrical impulses in cardiac and skeletal muscle. It plays a role in acid base equilibrium. In states of acidosis hydrogen with enter the cell as this happens it will force potassium out of the cell, a 0.1 decrease in pH will cause a 0.5 increase in K+.

What would cause increased levels?

acidosis, renal failure, diet, dialysis, burns, Addison's disease, ketoacidosis, trauma, hyperventilation, uremia

What would cause decreased levels?

CHF, alkalosis, hyperaldosteronism, toxic shock syndrome, malabsorption, excess insulin, Cushing's

Prealbumin

Normal

19-38 mg/dL

Indications

helpful in evaluating nutritional status

Description

protein produced by the liver, short half-life (2 days) making it a good indicator of protein status and malnutrition

What would cause increased levels?

steroid therapy, alcoholism

What would cause decreased levels?

malnutrition, chronic illness, inflammatory process, trauma, liver disease

Prostate Specific Antigen

Normal

Male: < 4 ng/mL
Female: < 0.5 ng/mL

Indications

utilized to evaluate enlarged prostate when prostate cancer is suspected, stage cancer, evaluate effectiveness of treatments

Description

PSA produced by prostate when used in conjunction with digital exam this test is helpful in diagnosing and assessing prostate abnormalities

What would cause increased levels?

BPH, prostate cancer, urinary retention

What would cause decreased levels?

N/A

Protein (total)

Normal

6 - 8 g/dL

Indications

diagnosing myeloma, lymphoma, macroglobulinemia, amyloidosis, evaluate kidney function

Description

Protein is an important contributor of energy in our diet. Protein has many numerous functions in the body

What would cause increased levels?

UTI, nephrotic syndrome, heavy metal poisoning, exercise, diabetic nephropathy, multiple myeloma, sickle cell disease, sarcoidosis, lymphoproliferative disorder

What would cause decreased levels?

N/A

Prothrombin Time

Normal

11 - 14 seconds

Indications

evaluate therapeutic doses of anticoagulants, identify patients at higher risk for bleeding, identify cause of bleeding, and deficiencies

Description

time it takes for a fibrin clot to form. Prothrombin is produced by the liver and is dependent on vitamin K.

What would cause increased levels?

disseminated intravascular coagulation, hereditary factors, liver disease, vitamin k deficiency, SLE, drug therapy,

What would cause decreased levels?

enteritis, ovarian hyperfunction

Red Blood Cell

Normal

Male: 4.5 - 5.5 $x10^6$/cells/mm^3
Female: 4.0 - 4.9 $x10^6$/cells/mm^3

Indications

helpful in identifying anemia, determine blood loss, part of the CBC and useful in a general physical exam.

Description

Red blood cells (RBCs) contain hemoglobin which is responsible for oxygen transport throughout the body. RBCs are primarily produced in the bone marrow, they have a life span of 120 days and are destroyed in the spleen and liver. RBC production is regulated by erythropoietin which is produced and released from the kidneys.

What would cause increased levels?

dehydration, polycythemia vera, COPD, bone marrow failure

What would cause decreased levels?

chemotherapy, anemia, hemorrhage, leukemia, organ failure, hypervolemia, pregnancy

Red Blood Cell Distribution Width

Normal

<14.5

Indications

Useful in the diagnosis of anemia

Description

Red blood cell distribution width (RDW) is a measurement of the variation of RBC cell size amongst the entire population of RBCs. Used with other red cell indices to determine cause of anemia.

What would cause increased levels?

Anemia, when combined with additional RBC indices specific cause for anemia can be better determined

What would cause decreased levels?

N/A

Sodium (serum)

Normal

135-145 mEq/L

Indications

the sodium ion is mostly found in the serum (extracellular) the test helps to evaluate total body sodium stores

Description

Sodium (Na) is the most abundant cation in extracellular fluid. Sodium aids in osmotic pressure, renal retention and excretion of water, acid-base balance, regulation of other cations and anions in the body, plays a role in blood pressure regulation, and stimulation of neuromuscular reactions. Generally speaking elevated sodium levels are often due to relative deficit of free water.

What would cause increased levels?

Cushing's disease, dehydration, burn injury, azotemia (elevated nitrogen), vomiting, lactic acidosis, fever, excessive iv fluids containing saline, diarrhea, diabetes,

What would cause decreased levels?

CHF, cystic fibrosis, diuretic use, metabolic acidosis, Addison's disease, nephrotic syndrome, excessive ADH, liver failure

Triglycerides

Normal

<150 mg/dL

Indications

evaluate for elevated triglycerides, estimate risk for atherosclerotic heart disease and stroke

Description

triglycerides are required to provide energy during the metabolic process, excess triglycerides are stored in adipose tissue

What would cause increased levels?

MI, alcoholism, anorexia nervosa, cirrhosis, HTN, nephrotic syndrome, obesity, renal failure, pancreatitis, stress

What would cause decreased levels?

COPD, liver disease, hyperthyroidism, malnutrition, malabsorption

Total Iron Binding Capacity

Normal

250-460 ug/dL

Indications

assess cause of anemia and whether anemia is associated with iron deficiency or another cause, assess iron metabolism and storage

Description

Total iron binding capacity is essentially a measure to determine if a patient has too much or too little iron in the body and how well iron is being transported

What would cause increased levels?

liver disease, iron-deficiency anemia, pregnancy

What would cause decreased levels?

infection, cirrhosis, protein depletion, renal disease

Troponin I

Normal

There is a wide range of normal values among varying institutions and texts with regard to Troponin I. It is essential to verify institutional norms.

< 0.035 ng/mL

Indications

evaluating damage to heart muscle, diagnose an MI

Description

Troponins are proteins that initiate contraction of muscle fibers. Troponin I is specific to heart muscle. Troponins stays elevated for a week after muscle damage then returns to normal.

What would cause increased levels?

heart damage, MI

What would cause decreased levels?

N/A

White Blood Cell

Normal

4,500 - 10,000 cells/mcL

Indications

white blood cells demonstrate the body's response or ability to respond to an infectious process

Description

White blood cells are created in the bone marrow, their primary function is to defend the body against infection. There are various types of WBCs which have different shapes and functions.

What would cause increased levels?

(leukocytosis) pregnancy, emotional stress, transfusion reaction, infection, Cushing's disease, leukemia (unnatural rise in immature WBCs)

What would cause decreased levels?

radiation, SLE, anemia, rheumatoid arthritis, viral infection

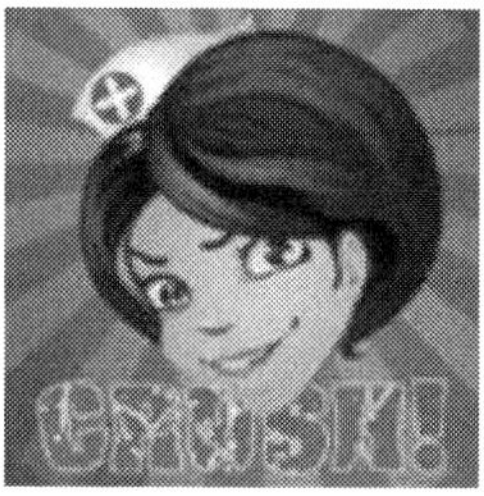

Introduction

Mnemonics and memory aids are one of the best ways for students to accelerate their learning.

This book contains 94 mnemonics specifically designed for nurses and nursing students preparing for the NCLEX® and who simply want to take their career to the next level.

The book is divided into sections based on nursing core content. With these mnemonics, colored pictures and detailed descriptions you will find yourself engaging and learning at a fast pace and retaining the information that you learn.

Be patient with yourself and take your time to learn the mnemonics that apply to the material you are currently learning or studying in school.

Learn more about our books at NursingStudentBooks.com or NRSNG.com. You can also contact me directly at contact@nrsng.com

Obstetrics/ Pediatrics

Cyanotic Defects

The 4 Ts

Tetralogy of Fallot
Truncus Arteriosus
Transposition of the Great Vessels
Tricuspid Atresia

Cyanotic heart defects are a group of congenital heart defects that result from deoxygenated blood by-passing the lungs and going into systemic circulation. Tetralogy of Fallot includes 4 anatomical abnormalities that are pictured below. Truncus Arteriosus is a condition where the pulmonary trunk and aorta don't properly divide in development. This results in one large vessel carrying mixed blood to the heart, lungs, and systemic circulation. Transportation of the Great Vessels is a condition where vessels or arteries are swapped or they may just be in abnormal positions. Tricuspid Atresia is a condition where there is no tricuspid valve which leads to undersized or absent right ventricle.

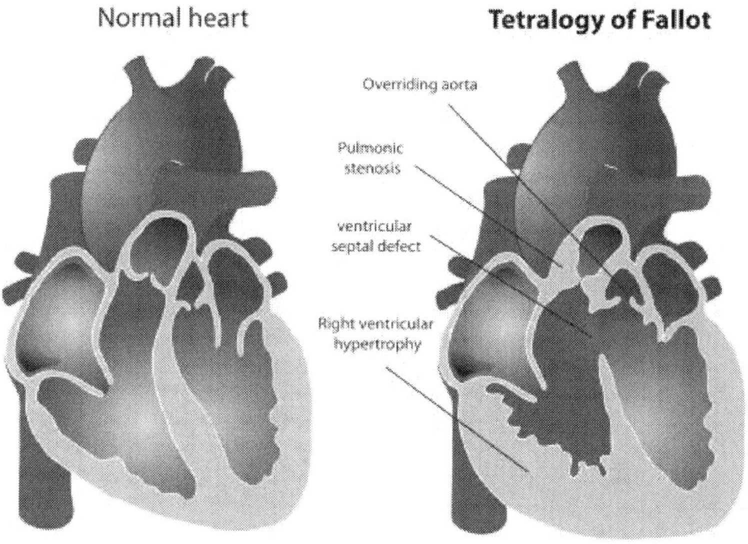
Normal heart
Tetralogy of Fallot
Overriding aorta
Pulmonic stenosis
ventricular septal defect
Right ventricular hypertrophy

Episiotomy- Evaluation of Healing

REEDA

Redness
Edema
Ecchymosis
Discharge, Drainage
Approximation

Redness with pain, excess edema, ecchymosis (bruising), or discharge from the wound can all be signs of problems with healing after an episiotomy. Wound edges should be well approximated. Topical ointments and ice packs may be indicated if there is pain or excess swelling, etc.

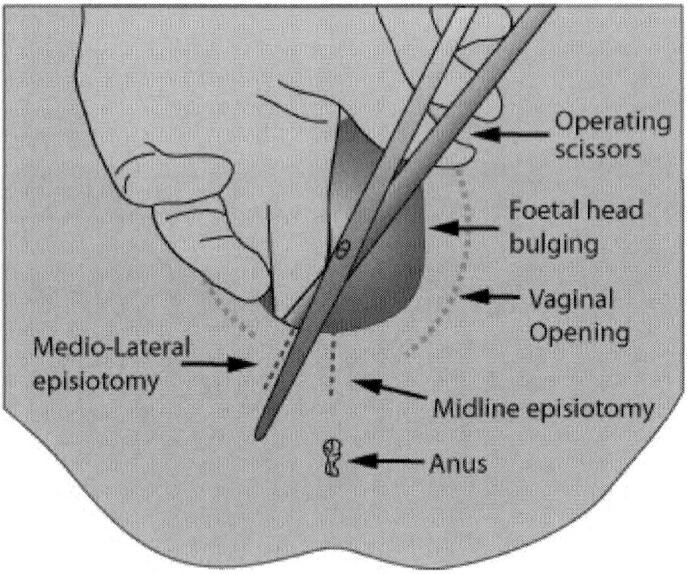

Fetal Accelerations and Decelerations

VEAL CHOP

Variable -	**C**hord Compression
Early -	**H**ead Compression
Accelerations -	**O**kay
Late -	**P**lacental Insufficiency

VEAL CHOP can be used to help remember how to interpret fetal heart rate during labor. For example early decels in FHR(fetal heart rate) indicate head compression. It is typical for decels in FHR during a contraction because of head compression, but FHR should return to normal when contraction ends.

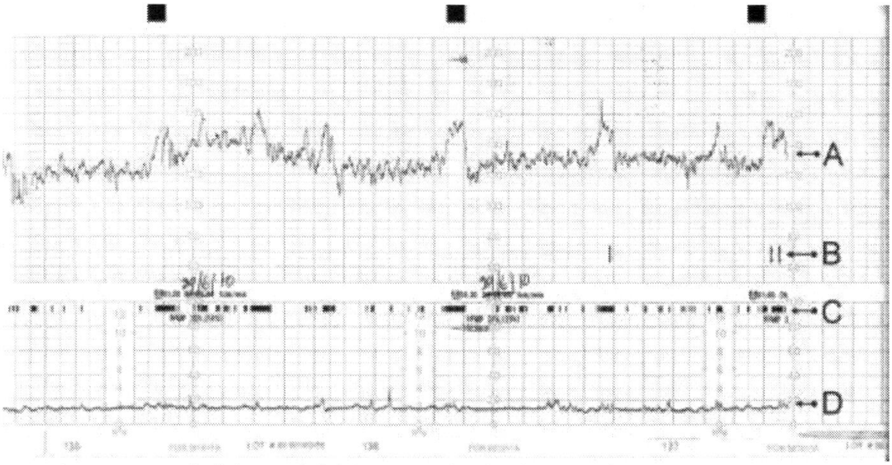

By -- PhantomSteve/talk|contribs\ (The original uploader was Phantomsteve at English Wikipedia) [CC BY-SA 3.0 (http://creativecommons.org/licenses/by-sa/3.0)], via Wikimedia Commons

Fetal Well-Being- Assessment Tests

ALONE

Amniocentesis
L/S Ratio
Oxytocin Test
Non-Stress Test
Estriol Level

An amniocentesis is preformed prenatally. A needle is inserted to obtain a sample of amniotic fluid. The fluid can be used to identify chromosomal abnormalities. L/S ratio compares lecithin–phosphatidyl choline to sphingomyelin to identify infant lung maturity. The oxytocin test measures fetal heart rate during contractions induced by oxytocin. A non-stress test measures fetal heart rate while baby is at rest and while baby is moving. Estriol levels in mother's blood can be a marker for fetal well-being.

Intra Uterine Device- potential problems with use

PAINS

Period (menstrual: late, spotting, bleeding)
Abdominal pain, dyspareunia (painful intercourse)
Infection (abnormal vaginal discharge)
Not feeling well, fever or chills
String missing

An intrauterine device is inserted into the uterus and is used to prevent pregnancy. There are two different types: hormonal and copper IUD.

OB Non-Stress Test -3 negatives in a row to interpret results of Non-Stress Test

NNN

Non-reactive
Non- Stress is
Not good

A non-reactive result in a non-stress is not good. During a non-stress test the fetal heart rate is monitored during movement. A reactive result is a good sign indicating intact central and autonomic nervous system. A reactive non-stress test result would be 2 accelerations to a certain level for greater than 15 seconds within a 20 minute period. If this does not occur the test is non-reactive.

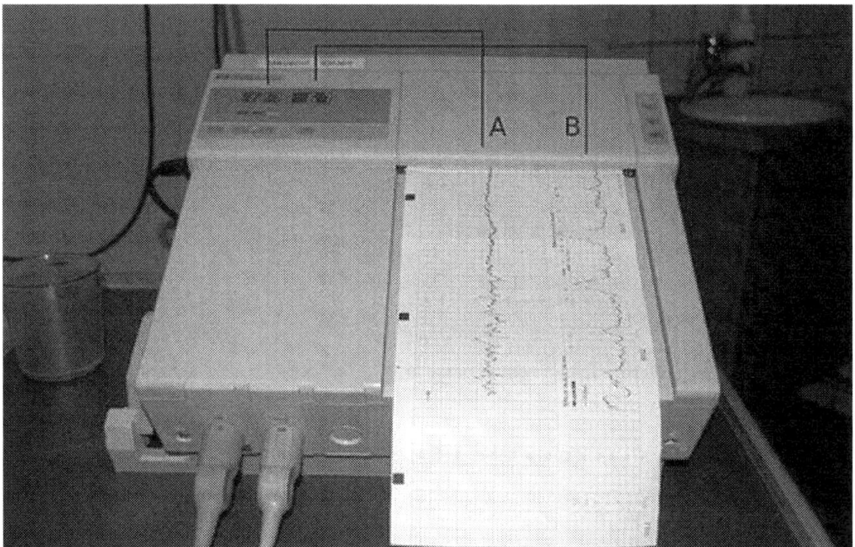

Oral Birth Control Pills- Serious Complications

ACHES

Abdominal Pain
Chest Pain
Headache
Eye Problems
Severe Leg Pain

Monitor for the following serious complications in patients taking oral contraceptives: abdominal pain, chest pain, headache, eye problems, swelling or aching in the legs or thighs.

Post-Partum Assessment

BUBBLE

Breasts
Uterus
Bowels
Bladder
Lochia
Episiotomy-laceration/C-section - incision

Make sure to assess the following in patients postpartum: 1. breasts - engorgement 2. Uterus -check the uterus for bogginess (firming up and dropping to original place 3. Bowel- flatus and bowel movement 4. Bladder – patient will likely have a catheter, check for anything unusual like blood in urine 5. Lochia – discharge 6. Episiotomy-laceration/C-section-incision – check for any signs that wound is not properly healing. (See acronym REEDA to assess episiotomy)

Severe Pre-Eclampsia- Signs and Symptoms

HELLP

Hemolysis
Elevated
Liver function tests
Low
Platelet count

HELLP syndrome is severe high blood-pressure. It typically occurs in the third trimester and usually is found in women that already have a diagnosis of pre-eclampsia. The defining characteristics are hemolysis (breakdown of red blood cells), elevated liver enzymes, and low platelet count.

Hypoxia- Signs and Symptoms (in Pediatrics)

FINES

Feeding difficulty
Inspiratory Stridor
Nares Flares
Expiratory Grunting
Sternal Retractions

The above signs are indications that the patient is attempting to draw in more oxygen. The patient will begin to compensate for the decreased tissue oxygenation by doing the above actions.

Child Abuse/Neglect- Warning Signs

CHILD ABUSE

Childs excessive knowledge on sex and abusive words
Hair growth in various lengths
Inconsistent stories from the child and parent/s
Low self-esteem
Depression

Apathy, no emotion
Bruised
Unusual injuries
Serious injuries
Evidence of old injuries not reported

Child abuse can be in many forms; physical, sexual, emotional, or neglect. Any act of commission or omission by a caregiver that harms or may cause harm to a child is child abuse. As a healthcare professional it is important to be in-tune with the preceding warning signs that can indicate child abuse.

Cleft Lip - Post Op Care

CLEFT LIP

Choking
Lie on back
Evaluate Airway
Feed Slowly
Teaching

Larger nipple opening
Incidence increases in males
Prevent crust formation and aspiration

Cleft lip is a slit in the skin above the lip. Typical treatment is reconstructive surgery. Post op care includes monitoring for choking. Baby will be positioned on back for sleeping to prevent trauma to sutures. Make sure airway is open and monitor for aspiration – baby should be in an upright position for feeding. Feed baby slowly with larger nipple opening. Prevent crust formation. Lastly provide education to parents regarding feeding and common concerns.

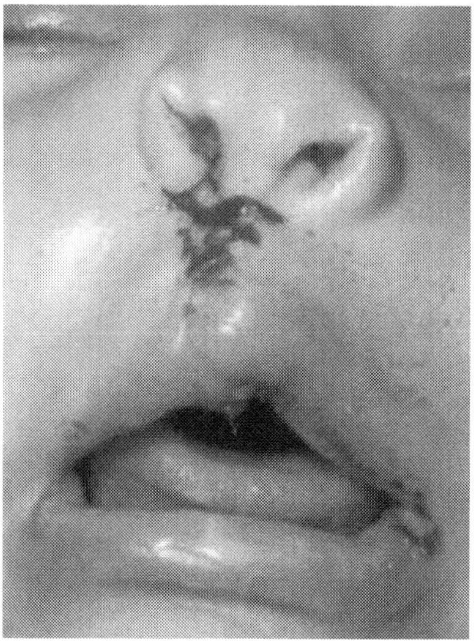

Tracheal Esophageal Fistula- Sign and Symptoms

The 3 Cs

Choking
Coughing
Cyanosis

A congenital abnormality in which there is an opening between the trachea and the esophagus. Surgery is required to repair the opening before a baby can receive po nutrition. Signs and symptoms to identify TEF (tracheal esophageal fistula) are choking, coughing, and cyanosis.

Labs

Hyperkalemia- Causes

The hyperkalemia MACHINE

Medications - ACE Inhibitors, NSAIDS, potassium-sparing diuretics
Acidosis - Metabolic and respiratory
Cellular destruction - burns, traumatic injury, hemolysis
Hypoaldosteronism (Addison's)
Intake- excessive
Nephrons, renal failure
Excretion - Impaired

Hyperkalemia is elevated potassium in the blood. Medications and kidney damage can decrease urinary excretion of potassium. In acidosis and cellular destruction potassium shifts from inside the cell to the blood stream. Excessive intake of potassium can also lead to hyperkalemia. Typical levels of potassium in the blood are 3.7 to 5.2 mEq/L.

Hyperkalemia- Signs and Symptoms

MURDER

Muscle weakness
Urine, oliguria, anuria
Respiratory distress
Decreased cardiac contractility
ECG changes
Reflexes, hyperreflexia, or areflexia (flaccid)

Potassium is necessary for the transmission of electrical impulses in heart and skeletal muscle. Potassium is also a part of reactions that breakdown glucose for energy. It can help maintain acid-base balance.

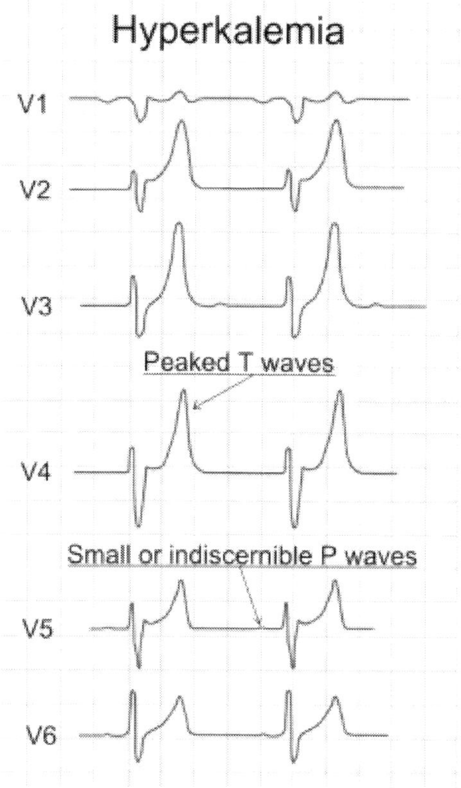
Hyperkalemia
V1
V2
V3
Peaked T waves
V4
Small or indiscernible P waves
V5
V6

Hyperkalemia- Management

KIND

Kayexalate (orally/ enema)
Insulin
Na HCO3
Diuretics (Furosemide & Thiazides)

The above treatments are utilized to reduce serum potassium levels. Kayexalate works by drawing potassium into the colon. Insulin increases cellular permeability to potassium. Sodium Bicarbonate (NaHCO3) works by increasing blood pH which in turn creates a shift of potassium into the cell as it shifts with the H ion moving out of the cell. Diuretics increase potassium wasting through the urine.

Hypernatremia- Signs and Symptoms

You are FRIED

Fever (low grade), flushed skin
Restless (irritable)
Increased fluid retention and increased BP
Edema (peripheral and pitting)
Decreased urinary output, dry mouth

Hypernatremia is elevated levels of sodium in the blood. Sodium helps with blood pressure and blood volume. It is also necessary for muscle and nerve function.

Hypernatremia- Signs and Symptoms

SALT

Skin flushed
Agitation
Low grade fever
Thirst

Hypernatremia is elevated levels of sodium in the blood. Sodium helps with blood pressure and blood volume. It is also necessary for muscle and nerve function.

Hypernatremia- Cause

MODEL

Medications /**M**eals

Osmotic diuretics

Diabetes insipidus

Excessive water loss

Low water intake

Hypernatremia is elevated levels of sodium in the blood. It can be caused by excess sodium intake or decrease in free water which leads to a higher concentration of sodium in the blood.

Hypernatremia- Management

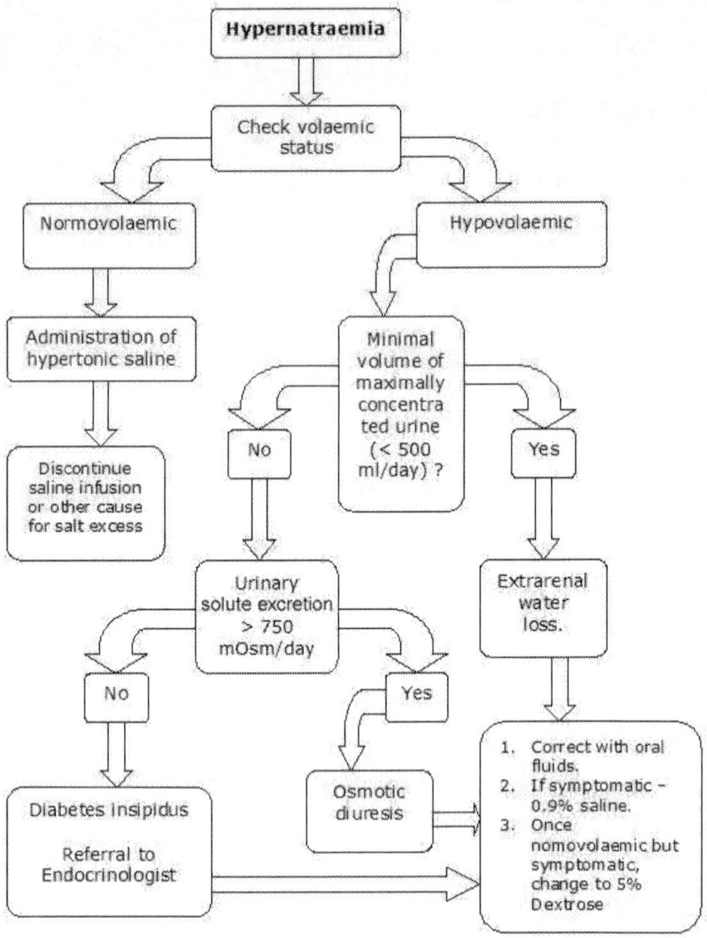

Hypernatremia may either be caused by too much sodium or too little water. First asses volume status of the patient then utilize the chart above to determine best course of action.

Hypocalcemia- Signs and Symptoms

CATS of hypocalcemia

Convulsions
Arrhythmias
Tetany
Spasms and stridor

Hypocalcemia is low levels of Calcium in the blood. Calcium in the blood can be bound to proteins, bound to anions like phosphate, or ionized. Large of stores of Calcium are in bone. Calcium blocks sodium channels, inhibiting depolarization of muscle and nerve fibers. The effects of hypocalcemia are a result of muscle fibers being more excitable

Hyponatremia- Signs and Symptoms

SALT LOSS

Stupor/coma
Anorexia, N&V
Lethargy
Tendon Reflexes decreased

Limp muscles (weakness)
Orthostatic hypotension
Seizures/headache
Stomach cramping

Hyponatremia is decreased levels of sodium in the blood. It can be caused by inadequate sodium or excess free water which leads to lower concentration of sodium. Sodium and Potassium work together to allow depolarization of muscles. Low sodium levels can limit this ability and cause muscle weakness. Sodium in the blood helps maintain the oncotic pressure. If fluid leaves the blood vessels that can lead to decreased blood pressure.

Hyponatremia- Signs and Symptoms

SALT LOSS

Stupor/coma
Anorexia, N&V
Lethargy
Tendon Reflexes decreased

Limp muscles (weakness)
Orthostatic hypotension
Seizures/headache
Stomach cramping

Hyponatremia is decreased levels of sodium in the blood. It can be caused by inadequate sodium or excess free water which leads to lower concentration of sodium. Sodium and Potassium work together to allow depolarization of muscles. Low sodium levels can limit this ability and cause muscle weakness. Sodium in the blood helps maintain the oncotic pressure. If fluid leaves the blood vessels that can lead to decreased blood pressure.

Electrolytes- Location in body

PISO

Potassium
Inside the cell
Sodium
Outside the cell

Potassium and Sodium are the two most abundant cations in the body and have an inverse relationship in regards to intracellular and extracellular concentrations. Potassium is primarily located within the cell and sodium is primarily located outside the cell.

Pharmacology

Beta 1 and Beta 2

Beta 1: heart
Beta 2: lungs
You have one heart and two lungs

Beta 1 adrenergic receptors are mostly found in the heart. Beta 2 adrenergic receptors are found in lungs, GI tract, vascular smooth muscle, skeletal muscle, liver. Beta 1 beta blockers act primarily on the heart. Beta 2 beta blockers act primarily on the lungs.

Drugs for Bradycardia & Low Blood Pressure

IDEA

Isoproterenol
Dopamine
Epinephrine
Atropine Sulfate

We are discussing here SYMPTOMATIC brady and low blood pressure. Bradycardia and hypotension are not necessarily adverse clinical findings in and of themselves.

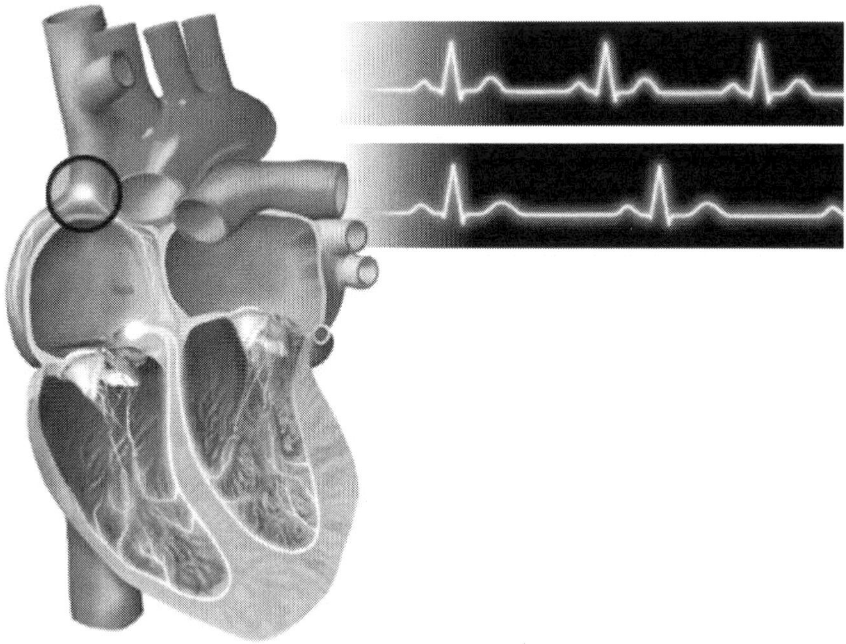

By Blausen Medical Communications, Inc. (Donated via OTRS, see ticket for details) [CC BY 3.0 (http://creativecommons.org/licenses/by/3.0)], via Wikimedia Commons

Drug Interactions

TDCI (These Drugs Can Interact)

Theophylline
Dilantin
Coumadin
Iosone (Erythromycin)

Coumadin and ilosone: ilosone can increase the effects of Coumadin, increase risk for bleeding.
Coumadin and Dilantin: potential for increase effects of both Coumadin and Dilantin
Theophylline and dilantin: if taken orally they can interfere with absorption of each other and decrease medication effect.

Emergency Drugs

Drugs to LEAN on

Lidocaine
Epinephrine
Atropine Sulfate
Narcan

The above drugs work in a variety of emergency settings. Lidocaine can be used in emergency situations for ventricular arrhythmias. Epinephrine is a vital drug in the ACLS protocol. Atropine can be given with symptomatic bradycardia and Narcan is a reversal agent for opiate overdose.

Lidocaine Toxicity

SAMS

Slurred Speech
Altered Central Nervous System
Muscle Twitching
Seizures

Lidocaine is an anesthetic that prevents painful impulses from reaching the brain. In the case of Lidocaine toxicity, look for slurred speech, altered central nervous system, muscle twitching, and seizures.

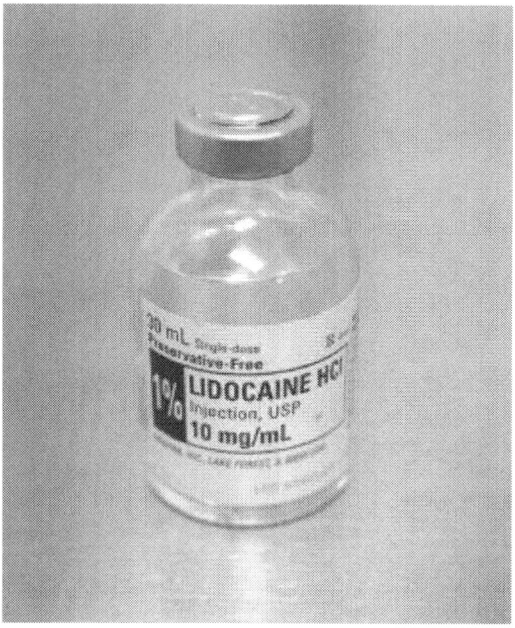

Steroid- Side Effects

6 Ss

Sugar-hyperglycemia
Soggy Bones - causes osteoporosis
Sick - decreased immunity
Sad - depression
Salt - water and salt retention (hypertension)
Sex - decreased libido

Steroids are an effective treatment for asthma, COPD, Crohn's, Lupus and more, however, they carry serious side effects. Steroids can be taken by mouth, via an inhaler, topically, or via injection. Side effects include elevation in blood sugars, elevation in blood pressure (due to water and salt retention), osteoporosis, depression, decreased libido, and decreased immunity.

Mental Health

Anorexia- Signs and Symptoms

ANOREXIA

Amenorrhea delayed
No organic factors accounts for weight loss
Obviously thin but feels FAT
Refusal to maintain normal body weight
Epigastric discomfort is common
X-symptoms (peculiar symptoms)
Intense fears of gaining weight
Always thinking of foods

Anorexia nervosa is an eating disorder characterized by low body weight and periods of starvation, or binging and purging. The lack of adequate nutrition and fat stores can lead to amenorrhea. Patients with anorexia will feel fat even if underweight; anorexia is an unhealthy way to cope with emotional problems. Binging and purging can lead to damage of the GI tract and epigastric discomfort. Some peculiar symptoms may also be seen: abnormal blood counts, bluish discoloration of the fingers, hair that thins, breaks or falls out, or soft downy hair covering the body.

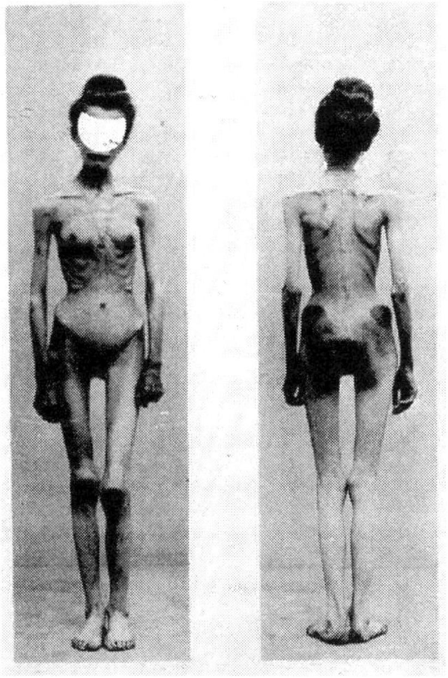

Bulimia- Signs and Symptoms

BULIMIA

Binge eating
Under strict dieting
Lacks control/over-eating
Induced vomiting
Minimum of two binge eating episodes
Increase/Persistent concern of body size/shape
Abuse of diuretics and laxatives

Bulimia is an eating disorder characterized by binging and purging. Patients may go through periods of excessive eating and then try to purge be inducing vomiting, taking laxatives or diuretics, or going through periods of fasting.

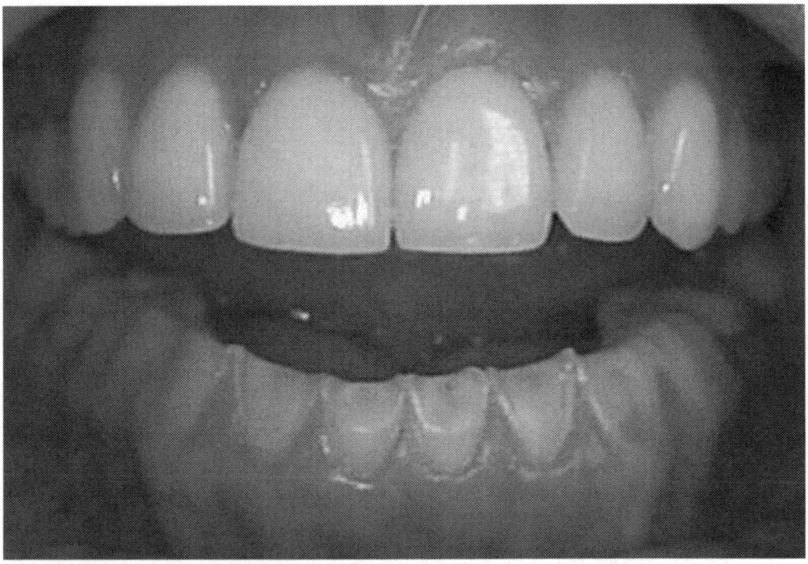

Bulimia- Signs and Symptoms

WASHED

Weight loss of 15% of original body weight
Amenorrhea
Social withdrawal
History of high activity & achievement
Electrolyte Imbalance
Depression/ Distorted Body Image

Alcoholism- Behavioral Problems

The 5 Ds

Denial
Dependency
Demanding
Destructive
Domineering

Abuse of alcohol can lead to very detrimental outcomes including those listed above. The preceding behavioral problems are common in people suffering from alcoholism.

Alcoholism- Outcome

BAD

Brain Damage
Alcoholic Hallucinations
Death

Abuse of alcohol can lead to very detrimental outcomes including those listed above. Emergent treatment should be provided for patients who have overdosed.

Depression Assessment

SIG

Sleep Disturbances
Interest Decreased
Guilty Feelings

Monitor for these signs and symptoms in patients that may be at risk for depression.

Manic Attack- Signs and Symptoms

DIG FAST

Distractibility
Indiscretion
Grandiosity

Flight of Ideas
Activity Increase
Sleep Deficit
Talkative

The above signs would be indicative of a patient experiencing a manic episode. A manic episode is a state in which the patient experiences abnormally elevated mood.

Alzheimer- Diagnosis

The 5 As

Amnesia – loss of memories
Anomia – unable to recall names of everyday objects
Apraxia – unable to perform tasks of movement
Agnosia – inability to process sensory information
Aphasia – disruption with ability to communicate

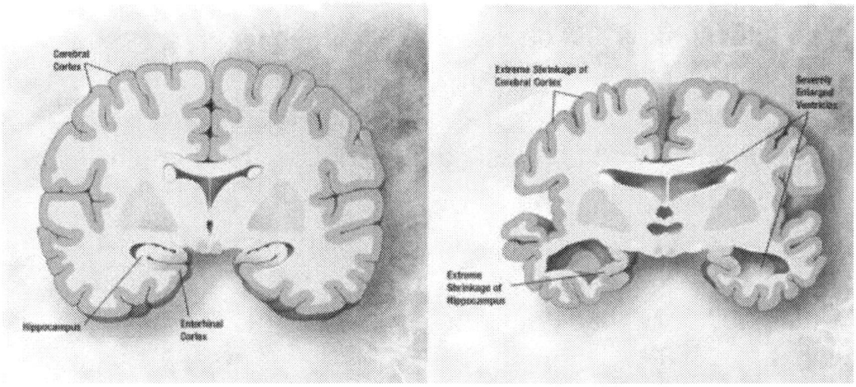

Dementia

DEMENTIA
Make sure they don't have problems with:

Drug and alcohol
Eyes and ears
Metabolic and endocrine disorders
Emotional disorders
Neurologic disorders
Tumors and trauma
Infection
Arteriovascular disease

When assessing a patient for dementia it is important to insure that one of the above listed conditions is an underlying cause for the dementia symptoms.

Senile Dementia- Assess for Changes

JAMCO

Judgment - can a patient determine the outcome of a choice, difficulty assessing risk
Affect - ability to express feeling or emotion
Memory - assess short and long term memory
Cognition- ability to process and relate information
Orientation- assess if a patient is oriented to person, place, time.

Med Surg

Arterial Blood Gases

ROME

Respiratory
Opposite
Metabolic
Equal

	pH	**pCO2**	**HCO3**	
Metabolic acidosis	Low	Normal	Low	Equal
Metabolic alkalosis	High	Normal	High	Equal
Respiratory acidosis	Low	High	Normal	Opposite
Respiratory alkalosis	High	Low	Normal	Opposite

First look at the pH: if it is low it is acidosis, high indicates alkalosis. Second use the ROME mnemonic to determine if you have respiratory vs. metabolic.

Pulmonary Edema- Treatment

MAD DOG

Morphine – causes vasodilation resulting in decreased BP
Aminophylline – relaxes airways to make breathing easier
Digitalis – improve heart function in pulmonary edema

Diuretics (Lasix) – pull excess fluid off
Oxygen – improve oxygenation
Gases (Blood Gases ABGs) – asses respiratory status

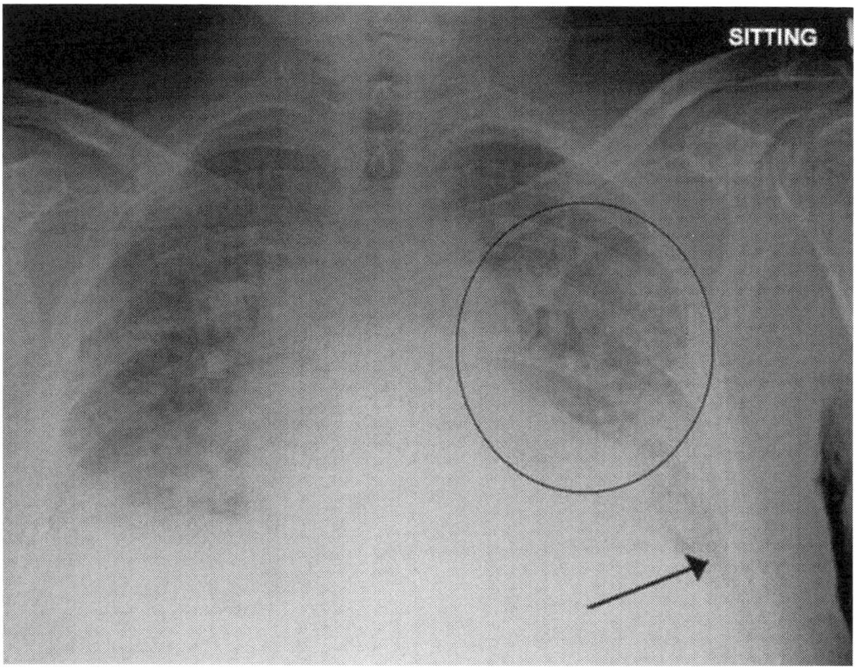

By James Heilman, MD (Own work) [CC BY-SA 3.0 (http://creativecommons.org/licenses/by-sa/3.0) or GFDL (http://www.gnu.org/copyleft/fdl.html)], via Wikimedia Commons

Dyspnea

The 6 Ps

Pulmonary Bronchial Constriction
Possible Foreign Body
Pulmonary Embolus
Pneumothorax
Pump Failure
Pneumonia

Bronchial constriction prevents the passage of air into the lungs which contributes to dyspnea. Foreign bodies can become trapped or logged within the trachea restricting air flow. PE can prevent complete oxygenation of the blood in the alveoli. Pneumothorax collapses the lung and prevents full expansion. Pump failure refers to the heart not beating appropriately. If the heart is not perfusing the lungs than the lungs will be unable to oxygenate the blood. Pneumonia leads to poor lung ventilation as well. These are six major causes for dyspnea.

Hypoxia- Signs and Symptoms

RAT BED

Early Hypoxia:
Restlessness
Anxiety
Tachycardia/ Tachypnea

Late Hypoxia:
Bradycardia
Extreme Restlessness
Dyspnea

Patients experiencing hypoxia will initially demonstrate signs of anxiety and restlessness. As hypoxia continues the patients conditions deteriorates to bradycardia and dyspnea.

Asthma- Management

ASTHMA

Adrenergic (Albuterol)
Steroids
Theophylline
Hydration (IV)
Mask (Oxygen)
Antibiotics

Asthma is a narrowing of the airways. It causes difficulty breathing. Medications can help open the airways.

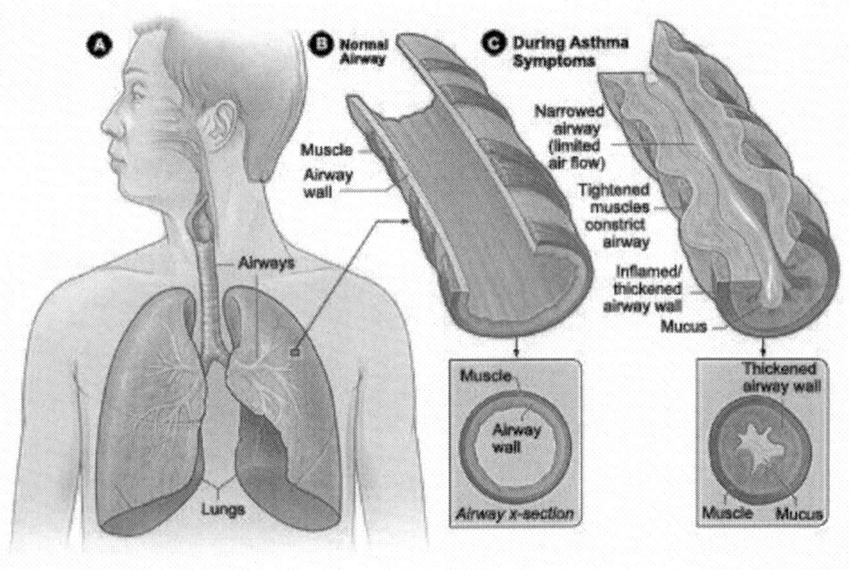

Pupillary reaction

PERRLA

Pupils
Equally
Round and
Reactive to
Light and
Accommodate

Under normal circumstances the pupils will be equally round. The pupils will dilate or constrict in dark or light respectively. The pupils will also accommodate when an item moves closer.

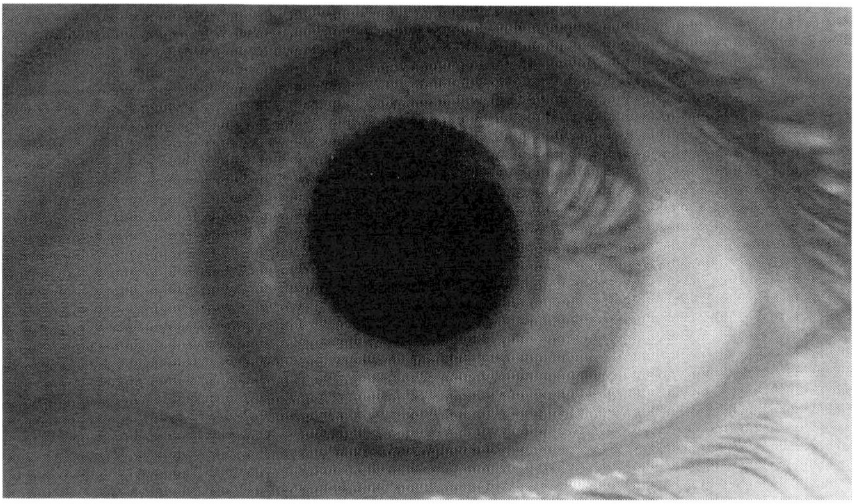

Moles- Malignant Potential

ABCD's

Asymmetry--is the mole irregular in shape?
Border--is the border irregular, notched, or poorly defined?
Color--does the color vary (for example, between shades of brown, red, white, blue, or black)?
Diameter--is the diameter more than 6 mm?

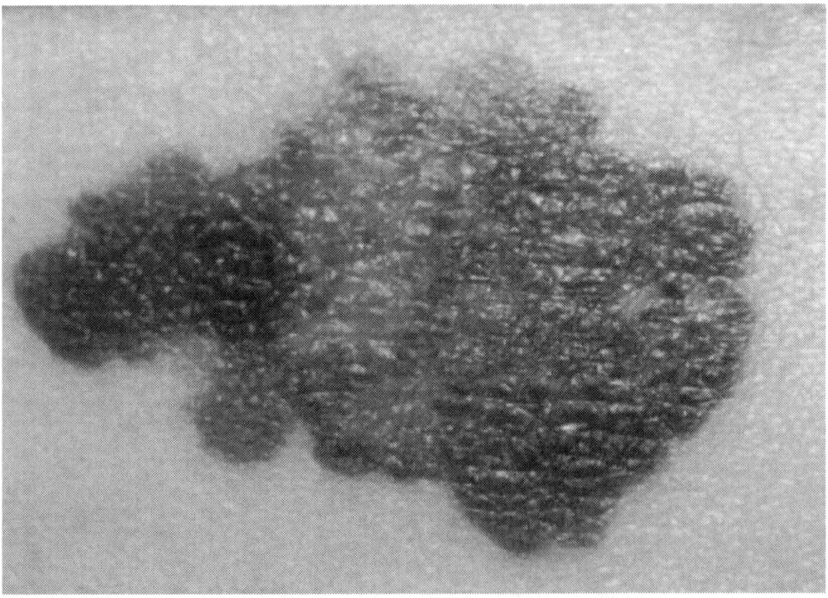

Diabetes Mellitus Type 1- Signs & Symptoms

The 3 Ps

Polyuria (excessive urination)
Polydypsia (excessive thirst)
Polyphagia (excessive hunger)

In type 1 diabetes mellitus a patient does not produce a hormone called insulin. Insulin allows sugar to go from the blood into the cells for energy. When sugar does not get into the cell sugar levels in the blood rise. The body tries to remove excess glucose by producing extra urine. The body then requires more water. We get hungry because our cells are starving for energy.

Hyperglycemia/Hypoglycemia

Hyper - hot/dry - sugar high
Hypo- cold/clammy - needs candy

During Hyperglycemia a patient is dehydrated, with elevated blood sugars. In hypoglycemia a patient is cold and clammy and need a carbohydrate source to bring their sugars back to a normal range.

Hypoglycemia- Signs and Symptoms

TIRED

Tachycardia
Irritability
Restless
Excessive Hunger
Diaphoresis/ Depression

During hypoglycemia the sugar (glucose) in the blood is too low. Cells of the body can't get adequate energy supply when there is not enough sugar in the blood. You will feel TIRED and have the symptoms listed above.

Circulatory Checks

The 5 Ps

Pain
Paresthesia
Paralysis
Pulse
Pallor (Paleness)

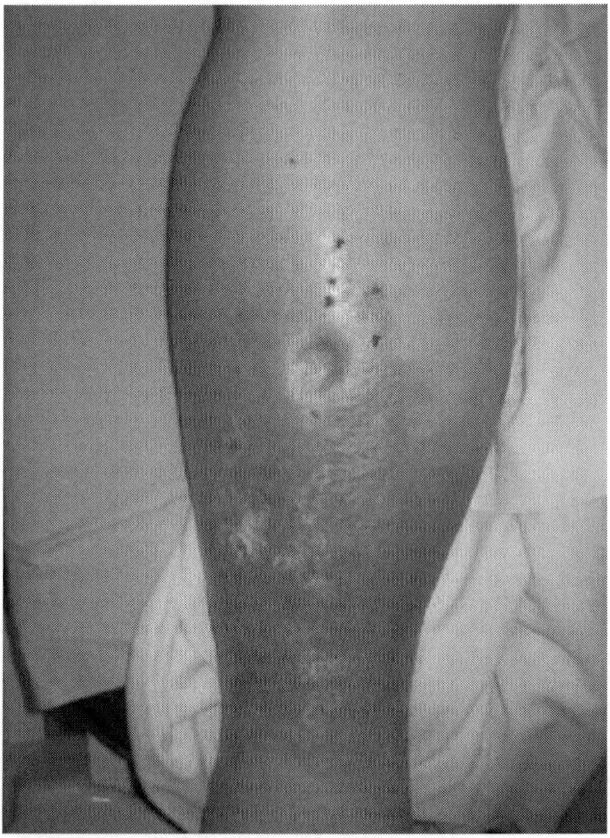

By James Heilman, MD (Own work) [CC BY-SA 3.0 (http://creativecommons.org/licenses/by-sa/3.0) or GFDL (http://www.gnu.org/copyleft/fdl.html)], via Wikimedia Commons

Hypertension- Nursing Care

DIURETIC

Daily Weight
Intake and Output (I & O)
Urine Output
Response of BP
Electrolytes
Take Pulses
Ischemic Episodes (TIA)
Complications: The 4 Cs on Hypertension (see next page)

For patients with elevated blood pressure monitor daily weights, intake and output, and urine output to watch for fluid retention. Monitor blood pressure and pulse in response to treatments. Diuretics may cause increase loss of electrolytes in the urine.

Hypertension- Complications

The 4 Cs

Coronary Artery Disease
Coronary Rheumatic Fever
Congestive Heart Failure
Cerebral Vascular Accident

Hypertension untreated can lead to vascular and valve destruction including those conditions listed above. Hypertension can also lead CVA or stroke in patients with long term uncontrolled hypertension.

Heart Sounds

APE To Man

Aortic
Pulmonic
Erbs points
Tricuspid
Mitral

This mnemonic is a great reference for cardiac auscultation.

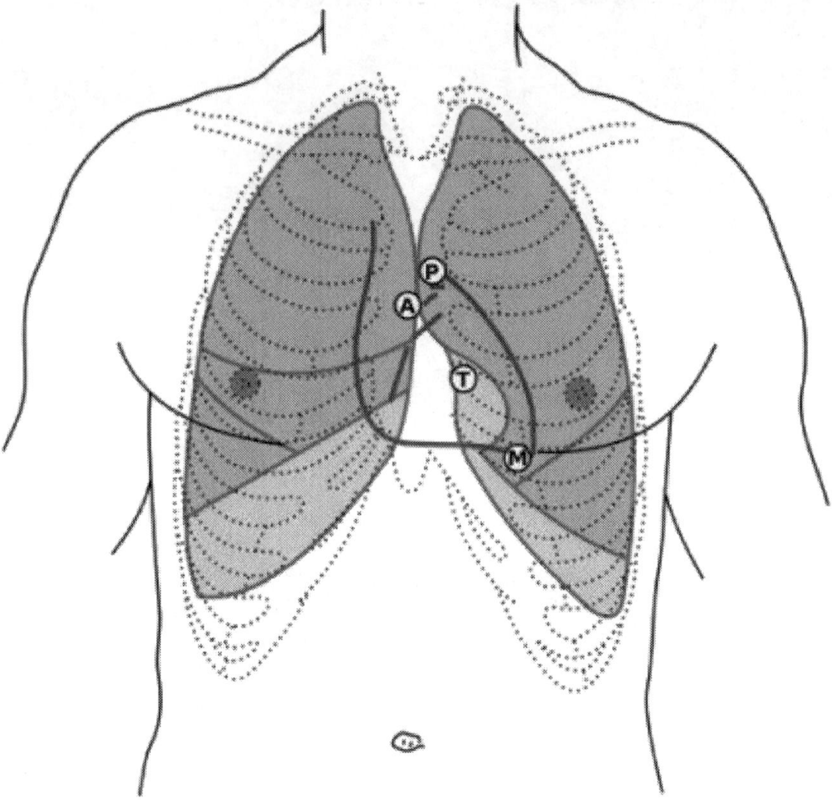
P
A
T
M

Cardiac Valves Blood Flow

Toilet Paper My A**

Tricuspid
Pulmonic
Mitrial
Aortic

This simple mnemonic helps to remember the order in which blood passes through the four heart valves in sequential order.

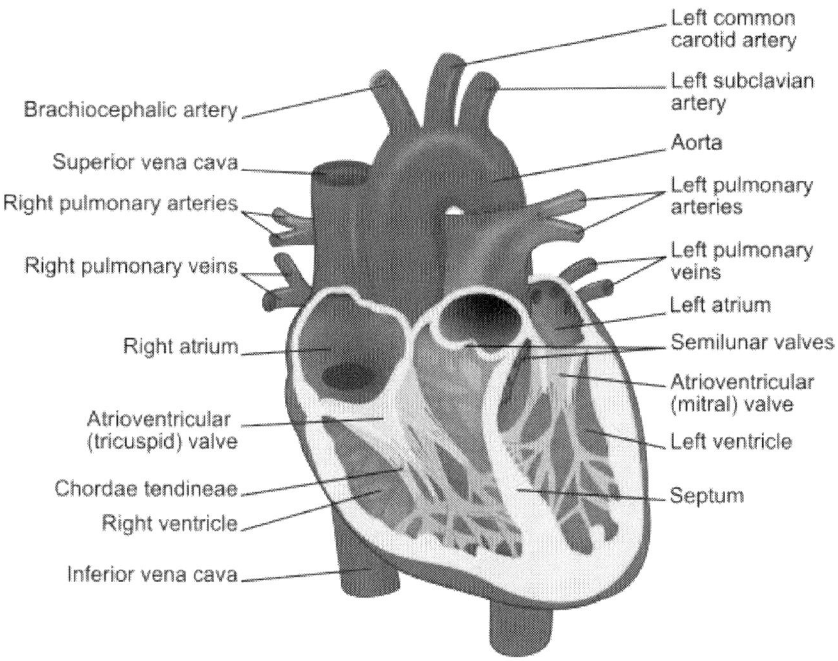

Myocardial Infarction- Immediate Treatment

MONA

Morphine sulfate
Oxygen
Nitroglycerin
ASA (aspirin)

After a myocardial infarction the immediate treatment is morphine sulfate, oxygen, nitroglycerin, and aspirin. Morphine works to decrease pain and difficulty breathing, oxygen insures that poorly oxygenated tissues receive the required O2, nitroglycerin is a potent vasodilator and aids in restoring oxygenation to tissues, aspirin helps to thin the blood and increase tissue perfusion.

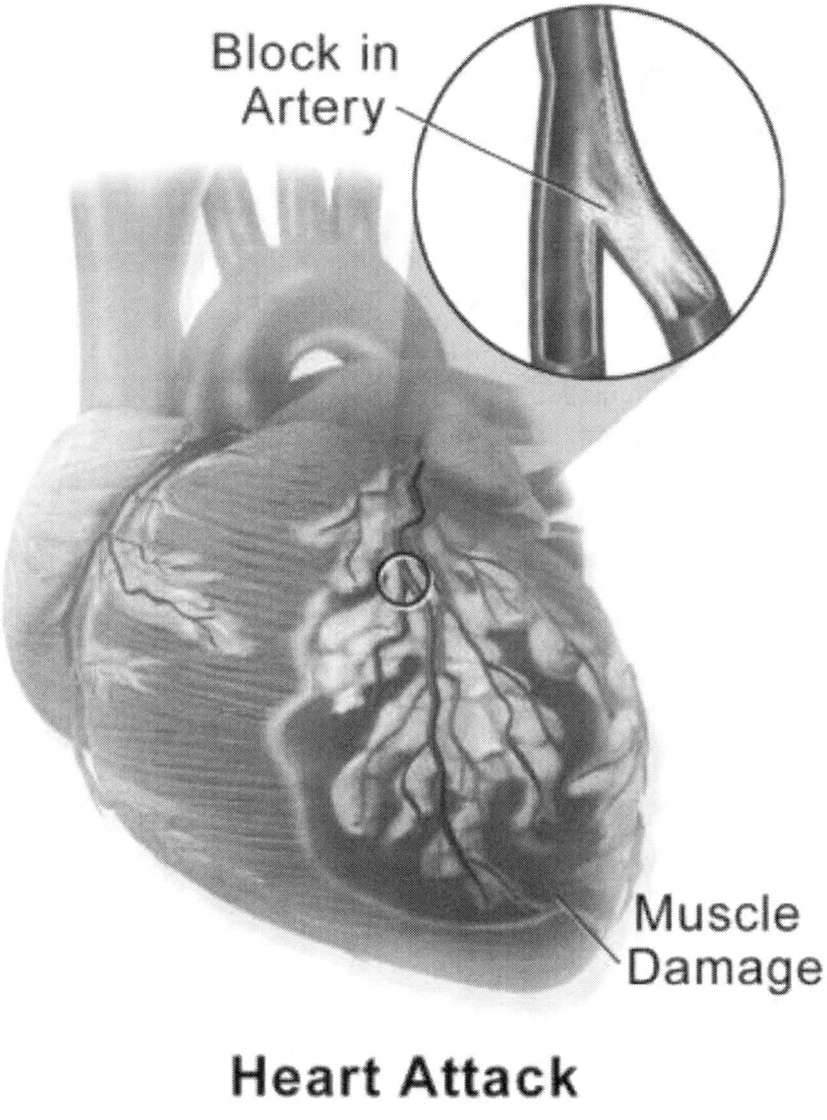
Block in
Artery
Muscle
Damage
Heart Attack

Myocardial Infarction- Management

MONATAS

Morphine
Oxygen
Nitrates (Nitroglycerin)
Aspirin (ASA)
Thormbolytics
Anti-Coagulants
Stool Softeners

Heart Failure- Right-Sided

HEAD

Hepatomegaly
Edema (Bipedal)
Ascites
Distended Neck Vein

Right sided heart failure will primarily manifest as central edema as the right side of the heart takes fluid from the body and moves it forward. If this portion of the pump is broken fluid will become "backed up" behind the pump . . . within the body.

Heart Failure- Left-Sided

CHOP

Cough
Hemoptysis
Orthopnea
Pulmonary Congestion (crackles/ rales)

Left sided heart failure will primarily manifest as pulmonary edema as the left side of the heart moves blood from the lungs throughout the body. If this portion of the pump is broken the blood will become "backed up" within the lungs. Left sided heart failure can often lead to right sided heart failure.

CHF- Treatment

UNLOAD FAST

U sit Upright
Nitro
Lasix
Oxygen
Aminophylline
Digoxin

Fluids - decrease
Afterload - decrease
Sodium - decrease
Tests: dig level, ABG, K+

These treatments used in conjunction will help in reducing the symptoms and complications associated with CHF.

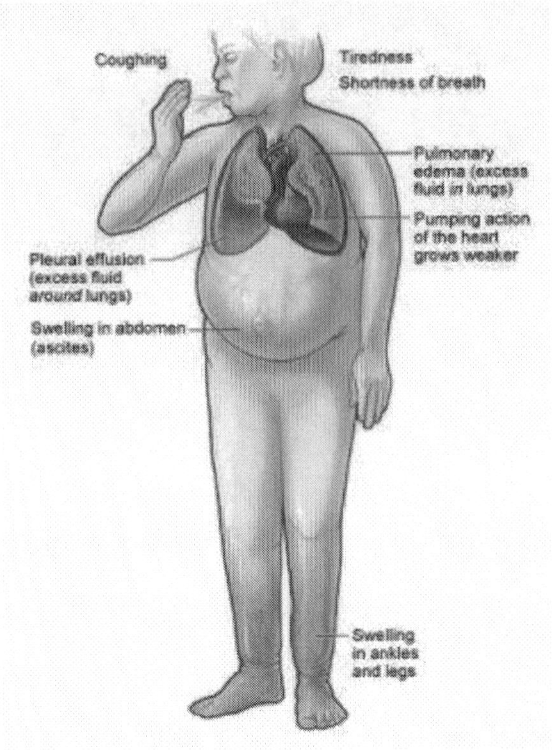
Coughing
Tiredness
Shortness of breath
Pulmonary edema (excess fluid *in* lungs)
Pumping action of the heart grows weaker
Pleural effusion (excess fluid *around* lungs)
Swelling in abdomen (ascites)
Swelling in ankles and legs

Inflammation- Signs and Symptoms

HIPER

Heat
Indurations (hardening)
Pain
Edema
Redness

In response to tissue damage the body elicits the inflammatory response in attempt to rid itself of the initial offender. These attempts can sometimes become more of a problem than a help.

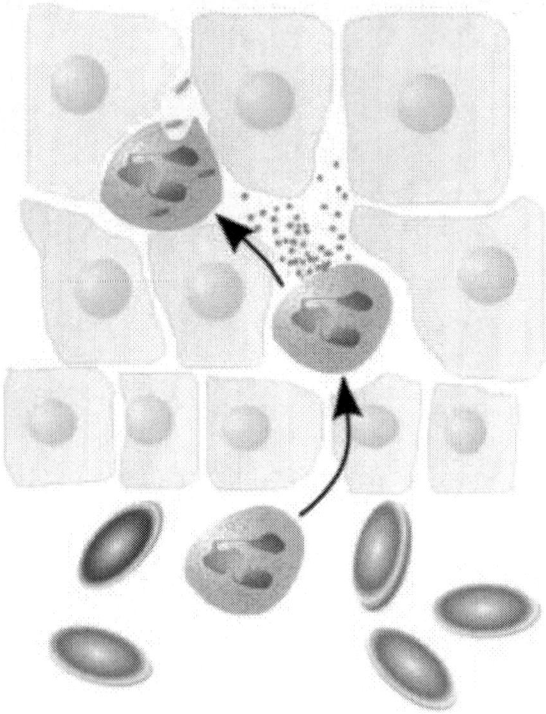

By Uwe Thormann (http://de.wikipedia.org/wiki/Benutzer:Uwe_Thormann) [GFDL (http://www.gnu.org/copyleft/fdl.html) or CC-BY-SA-3.0 (http://creativecommons.org/licenses/by-sa/3.0/)], via Wikimedia Commons

Toxicty/Sepsis- Signs and Symptoms

The 6 T's:

Tachycardia
Tachypnea
Tremors
Toxic look
Tiredness
Temperature (fever)

Sepsis is a systemic response to inflammation as a result of uncontrolled infection there is also a release of cytokines which lead to further inflammation and vascular dilation. Blood is shunted from the essential organs to non essential organs (the skin) leading to increased body temperature (along with response to infection). The heart begins to beat faster in response to the infection and to the decreased cardiac output as a result of the massive vasodilation.

Cancer- Early Warning Signs

CAUTION UP

Change in bowel or bladder
A lesion that does not heal
Unusual bleeding or discharge
Thickening or lump in breast or elsewhere
Indigestion or difficulty swallowing
Obvious changes in wart or mole
Nagging cough or persistent hoarseness

Unexplained weight loss
Pernicious Anemia

Cancer can sometimes be difficult to identify, but the earlier it is detected the better chance treatment will be effective.

Cancer- Interventions

CANCER

Comfort
Altered Body Image
Nutrition
Chemotherapy
Evaluate response to meds
Respite for caretakers

Leukemia- Signs and Symptoms

ANT

Anemia
Neutropenia
Thrombocytopenia

Leukemia can lead to anemia as it will disrupt the production of blood within the bone marrow. Neutropenia is a natural result of leukemia as the bodies supply of white blood cells is decreased. Thrombocytopenia is a reduced platelet count which can result from leukemia especially in infants.

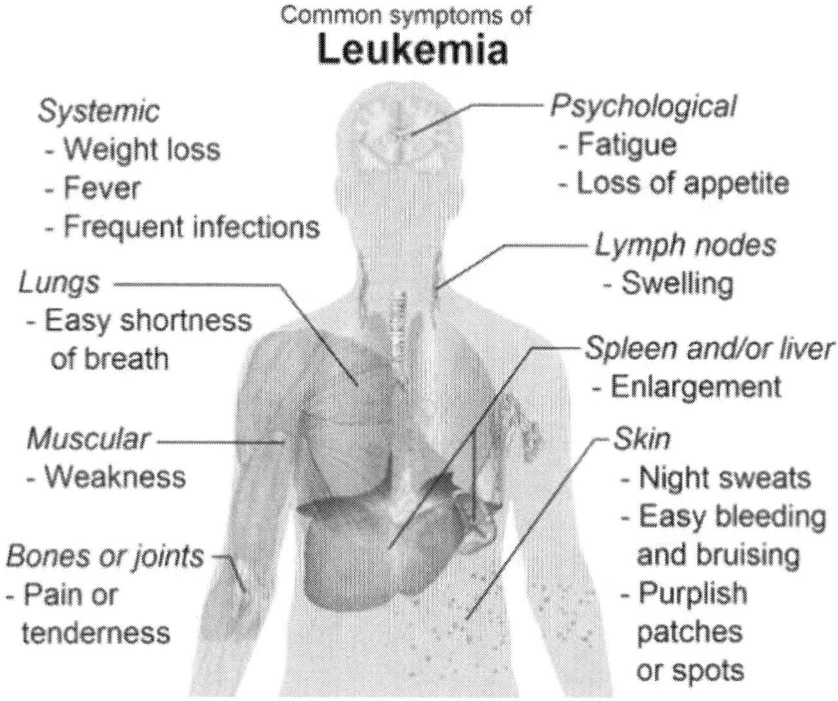
Common symptoms of
Leukemia
Systemic
- Weight loss
- Fever
- Frequent infections
Lungs
- Easy shortness of breath
Muscular
- Weakness
Bones or joints
- Pain or tenderness
Psychological
- Fatigue
- Loss of appetite
Lymph nodes
- Swelling
Spleen and/or liver
- Enlargement
Skin
- Night sweats
- Easy bleeding and bruising
- Purplish patches or spots

Appendicitis- Assessment

PAINS

Pain (RLQ) - pain in the right lower quadrant of the abdomen
Anorexia - loss of appetite
Increased temperature, WBC (15,000-20,000)
Nausea
Signs (McBurney's, Psoas)

> Psoas sign is pain when a patient extends their thigh while lying on their side with knees extended. It indicates irritation to certain muscles in the abdomen.
>
> McBurney's sign is if there is deep tenderness at mcBurney's point - right side of the abdomen, one-third the distance from the anterior superior iliac spine to the navel

Epiglottitis - Signs and Symptoms

AIR RAID

Airway Closed
Increased Pulse
Restlessness

Retractions- occur when the muscles between the ribs pull inward
Anxiety Increased
Inspiratory Stridor- high-pitched breath sound resulting from turbulent air flow in the larynx
Drooling

> The epiglottis is a flap of cartilage that covers the entrance to our airway when we swallow food. Inflammation of the epiglottis can close of the airway.

Cholinergic Crisis

SLUD

Salivation
Lacrimation
Urination
Defecation

A cholinergic crisis can occur if the body stops properly breaking down acetlycholine. This can cause an overstimulation of the neuromuscular junction.

COPD
- Ipratropium

Drugs to tx:

Myasthenia gravis
- edrophonium
- neostigmine

alzheimers
- rivastigmine
- donepezil

glaucoma
- pilocarpine

Adrenal Gland Hormones

The 3 Ss

Sugar (Glucocorticoids)
Salt (Mineralcorticoids)
Sex (Androgens)

There are three different adrenal gland hormones which can be remembered as the 3 Ss: sugar (Glucocorticoids) effect glucose utilization, fat metabolism and aid in reducing inflammation, salt (Mineralcorticoids) play a role in electrolyte regulation, sex (Androgens) commonly referred to as sex hormones.

Cranial Nerve Mnemonic 01

Olympic Opium Occupies Troubled Triathletes After Finishing Vegas Gambling Vacations Still High

Olfactory
Optic
Oculomotor
Trochlear
Trigeminal
Abducens
Facial
Vestibulocochlear
Glossopharyngeal
Vagus
Spinal Accessory
Hypoglossal

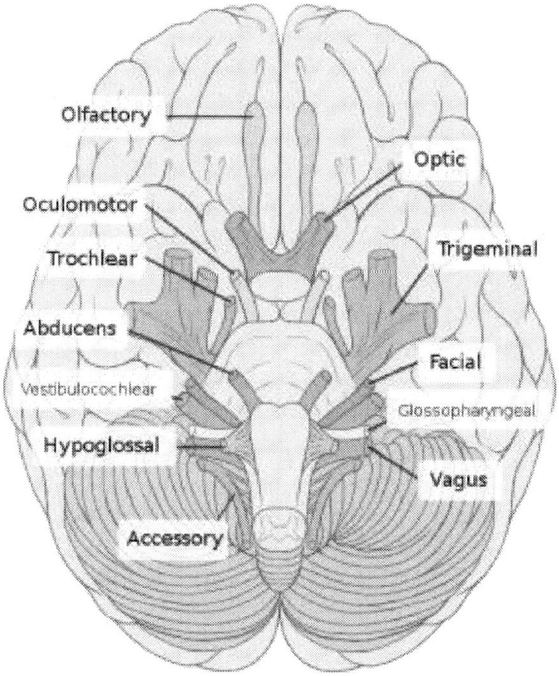

By Brain_human_normal_inferior_view_with_labels_en.svg:
*Brain_human_normal_inferior_view.svg: Patrick J. Lynch, medical illustrator derivative work: Beao derivative work: Dwstultz [CC BY 2.5 (http://creativecommons.org/licenses/by/2.5)], via Wikimedia Commons

Cranial Nerve Mnemonic 02

Oh Oh Oh To Touch And Feel Very Good Velvet AH!

Olfactory
Optic
Oculomotor
Trochlear
Trigeminal
Abducens
Facial
Vestibulocochlear
Glossopharyngeal
Vagus
Accessory
Hypoglossal

Cranial Nerve Mnemonic 03

On Old Obando Tower Top A Filipino Army Guards Villages And Huts

Olfactory
Optic
Oculomotor
Trochlear
Trigeminal
Abducens
Facial
Vestibulocochlear
Glossopharyngeal
Vagus
Accessory
Hypoglossal

Cranial Nerve Mnemonics- Sensory, Motor or Both

1: Some Say Marilyn Monroe But My Brother Says Bridget Bardot Mmm Mmm

2: Some Say Marry Money But My Brother Says Bad Business Marry Money

Olfactory	**S**ensory
Optic	**S**ensory
Oculomotor	**M**otor
Trochlear	**M**otor
Trigeminal	**B**oth
Abducens	**M**otor
Facial	**B**oth
Vestibulocochlear	**S**ensory
Glossopharyngeal	**B**oth
Vagus	**B**oth
Accessory	**M**otor
Hypoglossal	**M**otor

Prostate

Prostate Problems are no... FUN

Frequency
Urgency
Nocturia

As a patient begins to develop prostate issues they will start to demonstrate urinary symptoms including those listed above.

Diarrhea- treatment

Banana
Rice
Apple
Toast

The BRAT diet is a bland diet that is low in protein, fiber, and fat. It is thought to be easy on the GI tract and helpful to lesson diarrhea. It is not used commonly any more because of the lack of protein in the diet.

Transient Incontinence- Common Causes

DIAPPERS

Delirium
Infection
Atrophic Urethra- atrophy of the urethra
Pharmaceuticals- blood pressure medication, antidepressants, diuretics, sleeping pills
Psychologic
Excess Urine Output
Restricted Mobility
Stool Impaction

Promotion and Evaluation of Normal Elimination

POOPER SCOOP

(Promotion)
Position
Output
Offer Fluids
Privacy
Exercise
Report Results

(Evaluation)
Size (Amount)
Consistency
Occult Blood
Odor
Peristalsis

Bleeding Precautions

RANDI

Razor Electric/ Blades
Aspirin
Needles- small gauge
Decrease needle sticks
Injury (Protect from)

If a patient is taking an anticoagulant to prevent blood clots there is increase risk for bleeding. Be careful with blades when shaving. Do not take aspirin as it interferes with blood clotting and can magnify the effect of your medication. Avoid excess needle sticks and protect the patient from injury.

Trauma- Complications

TRAUMATIC

Tissue Perfusion Problems
Respiratory Problems
Anxiety
Unstable Clotting Factors
Malnutrition
Altered Body Image
Thromboembolism- fat embolism
Infection
Coping Problems

In trauma the patient needs to be quickly assessed for adequate perfusion as part of the trauma survey. Trauma can lead to overt or covert blood loss resulting in shock. If there is significant blood loss the patient may develop disseminated intravascular coagulation as they begin to deplete their available clotting factors.

Trauma- Assessment (Emergency)

ABCDEFGHI

Airway
Breathing
Circulation
Disability
Examine
Fahrenheit
Get Vitals
Head to Toe Assessment
Intervention

Rapid assessment and treatment of the trauma patient is essential to their overall survival. Working through this framework will aid in remembering where to focus your efforts. Always remember your ABC and patient safety. Once those things have been secured you can move on to less vital components.

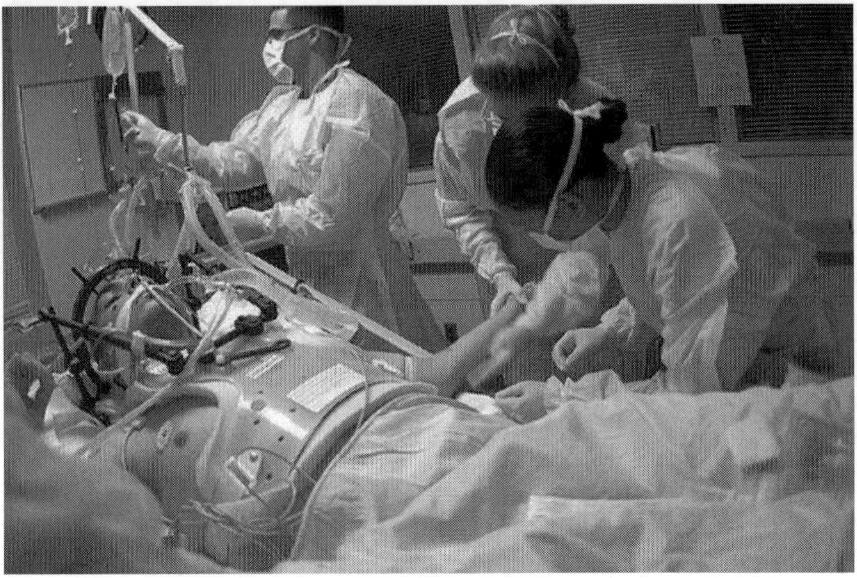

Trauma Surgery- After initial assessment

AMPLE

Allergies
Medications
Past Medical History
Last Meal
Events Surrounding Injury

Exercise Guidelines

FIT

Frequency (3x per week)
Intensity (60-80% of Maximal Heart Rate)
Time (Aerobic Activity)

Osteoporosis- Risk Factors

ACCESS

Alcohol Use
Corticosteroid Use
Calcium low
Estrogen low
Smoking
Sedentary lifestyle/s

ACCESS leads to OSTEOPOROSIS

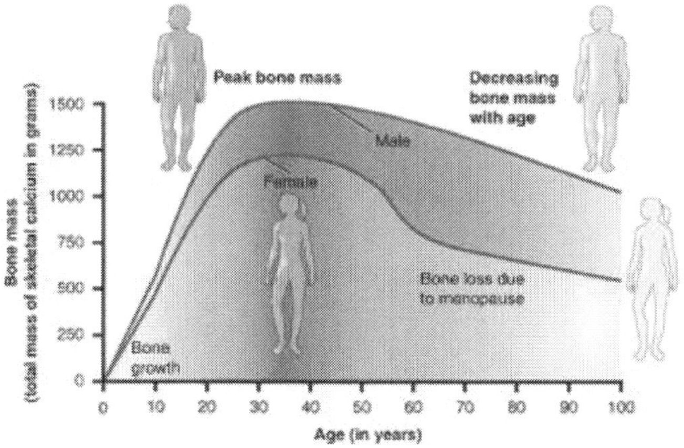

By Anatomy & Physiology, Connexions Web site. http://cnx.org/content/col11496/1.6/, Jun 19, 2013. (OpenStax College) [CC BY 3.0 (http://creativecommons.org/licenses/by/3.0)], via Wikimedia Commons

Dialysis- Who needs dialysis?

Check the vowels: AEIOU

Acid-Base Problems
Electrolyte Problems
Intoxications
Overload of fluids
Uremic Symptoms

As a patient progresses from chronic kidney disease to end stage renal disease the need for dialysis becomes more imminent. When the kidneys are no longer able to filter the blood alone you will see problem metabolic acidosis since they kidneys can't excrete excess acids that are in the blood. During kidney failure excess potassium isn't excreted and levels will start to rise. The kidneys help remove certain medications from the body, and when they aren't working toxicity can occur even with normal doses. Patients with ESRD become fluid overloaded due to inadequate urine production. Uremia will occur as the body can't excrete enough urea.

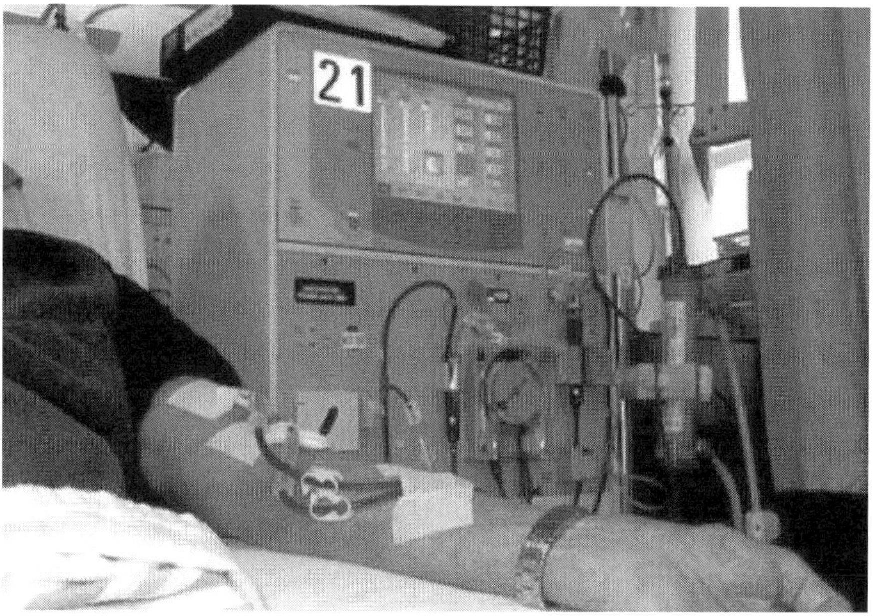
21

Gluten Free Diet

BROW

Barley
Rye
Oats
Wheat

Gluten is a protein found in wheat, barley and rye. People with gluten allergies can be affected by even trace amount of gluten in foods. Oats do not contain gluten, but they are often milled in the same factories as wheat. Always check food labels to make sure a product is gluten free

Nursing Fundamentals

Body Systems

MR DICE RUNS

Muscle
Respiratory

Digestive
Integumentary
Circulatory
Endocrine

Reproductive
Urinary
Nervous
Skeletal

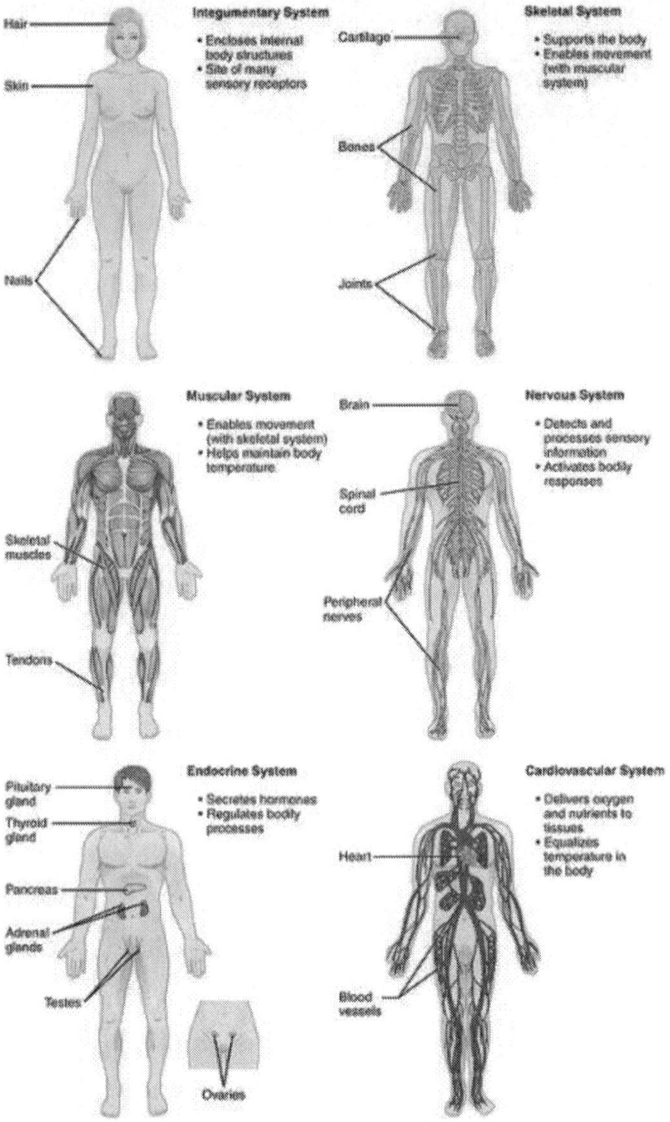
Integumentary System
• Encloses internal body structures
• Site of many sensory receptors
Hair
Skin
Nails
Skeletal System
• Supports the body
• Enables movement (with muscular system)
Cartilage
Bones
Joints
Muscular System
• Enables movement (with skeletal system)
• Helps maintain body temperature
Skeletal muscles
Tendons
Nervous System
• Detects and processes sensory information
• Activates bodily responses
Brain
Spinal cord
Peripheral nerves
Endocrine System
• Secretes hormones
• Regulates bodily processes
Pituitary gland
Thyroid gland
Pancreas
Adrenal glands
Testes
Ovaries
Cardiovascular System
• Delivers oxygen and nutrients to tissues
• Equalizes temperature in the body
Heart
Blood vessels

Steps in the Nursing Process

ADPIE (A Delicious PIE)

Assessment
Diagnosis
Planning
Implementation
Evaluation

Steps in the Nursing Process

AAPIE (An Apple PIE)

Assessment
Analysis
Planning
Implementation
Evaluation

Sprains and Strains- Nursing Care

RICE

Rest
Ice
Compression
Elevation

Traction- Nursing Care

TRACTION

Temperature (Extremity, Infection)
Ropes hang freely
Alignment
Circulation Check (5 Ps)
Type & Location of fracture
Increase fluid intake
Overhead trapeze
No weights on bed or floor

ADLs (Activity of Daily Living)

BATTED

Bathing
Ambulation
Toileting
Transfers
Eating
Dressing

When assessing a patient's ability to care for themself at home we must assess their ability to complete activities of daily living. A patient's ability to bath, walk, and toilet on their own will help us determine the level of care they will need when they leave the hospital.

IADLS (Instrumental Activities of Daily Living)

SCUM

Shopping
Cooking and Cleaning
Using telephone or transportation
Managing money and medications

The instrumental activities of daily living are used to determine a patient's ability to carry out necessary functions for independent living. If they are unable to manage the activities above, they will likely require some sort of assistance from family or a home health agency, etc.

Canes

COAL

Cane
Opposite
Affected
Leg

When teaching a patient how to walk with a cane it is important to instruct them to keep the cane on the opposite side of the affected extremity.

Walkers

Wandering Wilmas Always Late

Walker
With
Affected
Leg

When walking with a walker the patient should lift the walker as they lift their affected leg. This allows for the "good" leg to support the movement of the walker.

About the Authors

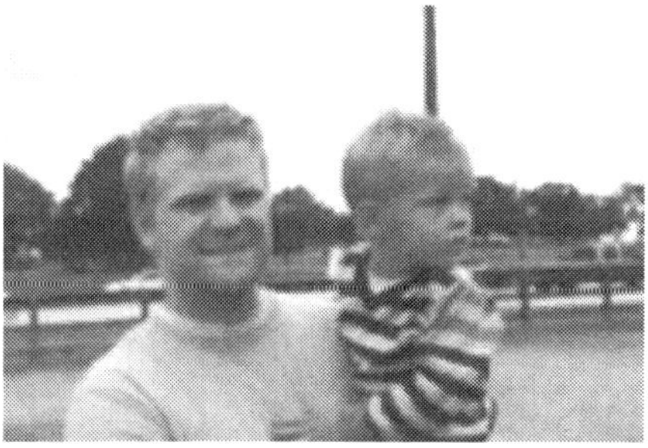

Sick of spending hours and hours trying to find all the information you need for clinical and NCLEX® study? So was I . . . . That's why I created NRSNG.com, a community of nurses and nursing students wanting to jump start their careers.

I am a registered nurse and CCRN on a Neurovascular Intensive Care Unit at a Level I Trauma Hospital. I attended college at Brigham Young University and later received my Nursing degree from Methodist College in Peoria, IL. I also hold a Business Management degree from Touro University.

Professionally, I precept nursing students and new graduate Registered Nurses and work as a charge nurse . . . and love it!

Come visit us at NRSNG.com or check in on Facebook.com/NRSNG

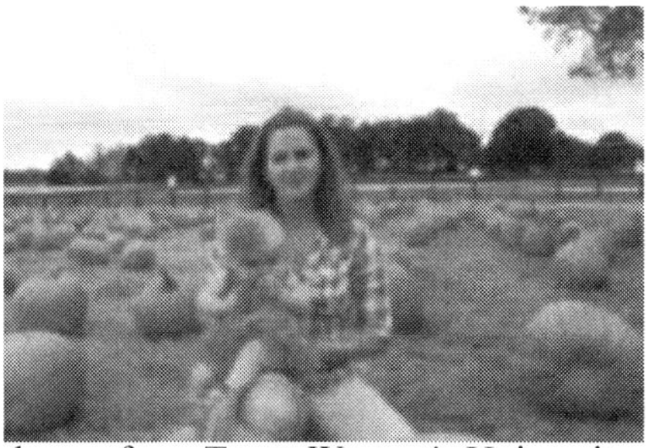

Sandra is a dietitian with one of the largest health care systems in the United States. She works with intensive care patients. She obtained her undergraduate degree from Brigham Young University and her graduate degree from Texas Woman's University. She holds advanced certifications in nutrition support management.

Your Free Gift!

As a way of saying thanks for your purchase, I'm offering a free PDF download:

"63 Must Know NCLEX® Labs"

With these charts you will be able to take the 63 most important labs with you anywhere you go!

You can download the 4 page PDF document by going to NRSNG.com/labs

Reviews greatly help this book reach more students. If you enjoyed this book please leave a review on Amazon or share the book on Facebook. Nothing helps more than a few kind words.

29768497R00310

Made in the USA
San Bernardino, CA
27 January 2016